T0154838

THE
HAPPY,
HEALTHY
REVOLUTION

THERESA Y. WEE, M.D.

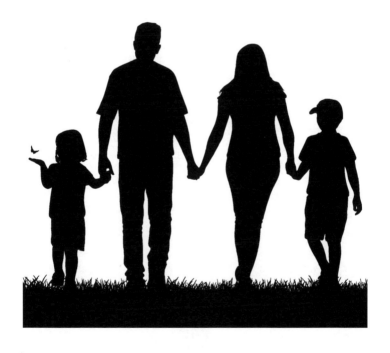

THE WORKING PARENT'S GUIDE TO
ACHIEVE WELLNESS AS A FAMILY UNIT

THE HAPPY, HEALTHY REVOLUTION
The Working Parent's Guide to Achieve Wellness as a Family Unit

Difference Press, Washington, D.C., USA
© Theresa Wee, 2021

ISBN: 978-1-68309-292-6

Cover Design: Nakita Duncan
Interior Book Design: Anna Zubrytska
Editing: Nkechi Obi

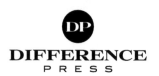

ADVANCE PRAISE

"As a friend and colleague for twenty years, I know that Theresa practices what she preaches. *The Happy, Healthy Revolution* doesn't just identify America's problems of obesity and family dysfunction, but more importantly demonstrates practical ways to solve them. If you put into practice what she preaches, it will lead to a healthy, well balanced lifestyle that will bring joy to you and your family each day."

– John H. Houk, MD, FACP, John A. Burns School of Medicine Assistant Clinical Professor

"Theresa's holistic approach to wellness is both refreshing and effective. It is grounded in personal experience and perfectly reflects Hawaii values. This book should be considered a roadmap to good health for families nationwide."

– Josh Green MD, Hawaii Lieutenant Governor

"It is an honor to have supported Theresa Y. Wee MD through AlohaCare's Waiwai Ola Community grant in the recent year! As a Hawaii pediatrician, she has been caring for our keiki and families, and her expertise has impacted her approach to preventing and treating obesity in Hawaii through an innovative family approach. *The Happy Healthy Revolution* is based on Dr. Wee's Family Workshops from the Waiwai Ola Grant. Her plan for healthy living helps people to see that each day counts."

– Carol Sato, AlohaCare Care Strategy Director

"Dr. Theresa Wee walks beside us, sharing her life's journey and weaving insightful expertise and sage guidance in *The Happy, Healthy Revolution*. If you ever felt alone or discouraged as a parent – hang on – hope is here.

– Danny Yamashiro, Radio Host of The Good Life Hawaii 99.5 KGU-FM

"Growing up in Hawaii, Dr. Wee embraced 'working hard' as one of her core values from her family of origin. In *The Happy, Healthy Revolution*, she exposes how the same will can sometimes threaten family values. From her own experience, Dr. Wee offers insights on how to balance 'doing' and 'being' in order to achieve a sense of well-being. The most practical and most valuable piece of work for our much-needed present context."

– Rev.JP Sabbithi, D.Min Pastor, Joy of Christ Lutheran Church, Pearl City, Hawaii.

For Stephen L. Wee. MD

You are so loved and so missed, but your legacy of compassion and service to others lives on. Thank you for being such a wonderful husband, father, and physician. You have positively touched and changed so many lives in your brief lifetime.

TABLE OF CONTENTS

FOREWORD

When Dr. Wee shared she was writing a book, I told our Walk with a Doc team, "This is fantastic. This is exactly who should be sharing how it is done!" Then, she asked if I would be willing to write the foreword. It is an honor. After reading the final product, I was, once again, so proud of Theresa. She has nailed something that is so critically important to us all.

I first came to know Dr. Wee in 2013 through introductions of mutual friends. She eventually started her own chapter of Walk with a Doc on Oahu about five years ago and has been impressing us nonstop since. Her chapter and her legend continue to grow.

Dr. Wee gets "it." As individuals, we all have the power to prevent, treat, or cure so many of the problems that can interrupt our daily lives. Yet, often we need someone to guide us through that tunnel. Dr. Wee does that for us.

Theresa's passion for others is on grand display as she leads us through the ins and outs of getting those simple, small wins that all add up to change our lives in a big, big way. I am so grateful that Dr. Wee took the time to share with us all what has made her a raging success with her patients, their families, and her community.

Nothing is more important than our health. Theresa, thank you from the bottom of my heart for being such a beacon of light and getting it all down in this wonderful book. You are a gift to us all!

With great respect,

David Sabgir, M.D. Cardiologist
C.E.O. and Founder – Walk with a Doc

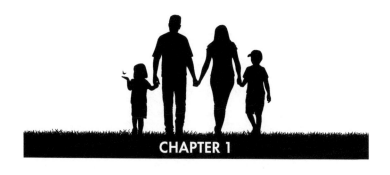

CHAPTER 1

FAMILY HEALTH IN JEOPARDY

As a young girl growing up in Hawaii in the sixties, I believed in fairy tales, happy endings, and dreams always coming true. My parents told me that I could be anything I wanted to be, and the world was bursting with great opportunities, even for women. Although my mom was a licensed social worker with a master's degree, she chose to be a stay-at-home mom after having all four of us children. I was determined to have it all.

At the tender age of seven years old, after reading an autobiography of the first woman to become a doctor, Elizabeth Blackwell, I discovered my calling in life. In the sixties, there were only a few women physicians in Hawaii, but her story truly inspired me. In addition to wanting to be a doctor, I also wanted to be married and have a family of my own, preferably with four children.

THE STRUGGLES OF WORKING MOTHERS

As the years unfolded, and with a lot of hard work, effort, and perseverance, I accomplished these goals, even the part about having four children. As a full-time, practicing pediatrician and working mom, I found out very quickly that I too was struggling to juggle the constant demands and details that come with working both in the home and outside the home. Even though "women's liberation" and equal rights were big topics, childcare and household matters still seemed to be the responsibility of women.

Early in my pediatric practice, I witnessed working mothers stretched to the limit, chronically tired, and trying their best to make it work both inside and outside the home. They had no time to buy groceries or prepare a healthy meal every night. Instead, they defaulted to fast food or takeout pizza, then wrestled with a guilty conscience for the rest of the evening.

The weekends are the time for these mothers to finally catch up on all the household chores, but unfortunately, this leaves no time for the mother herself, the husband, or the family. Dad, in the meantime, is also busy with his "Dad duties," like yardwork, house repairs, "honey-do lists," or working his second, part-time job. As a result, husbands and wives have no time to connect with one another or their children. They end up both feeling stressed to the max, and they each feel as if they are doing their best just to survive the week.

Every day in the office, I personally witness this lack of time for recharging ultimately result in many marriages eroding, children with behavior and mental health problems, and confusion and chaos within the family unit. Initially, as a young pediatrician, I was shocked to see how small disagreements over time slowly added up to monumental challenges and conflict within the family.

In medical school and residency training, I was thoroughly instructed about physical illnesses, diseases, treatments, and medications, but I was not prepared to address the many challenges families, parents, and children were starting to face in this new era of technology, fast foods, mental illness, and social isolation.

As the years went on, I found that as newer and more effective vaccines became available, I was no longer seeing as many critically ill children as I had during my pediatric residency training in the early eighties. Admitting children to our pediatric hospital was soon becoming a rare event, but now a new epidemic is starting to take its place. I am now witnessing the slow dissolution of the family unit. Family conflicts, dysfunction, and breakups are becoming more and more common.

NEW EMERGING TREND OF OBESITY IN ALL AGES

One of the first concerning trends I noticed was the rapid rise of more and more children becoming overweight or obese. They were slowly developing unhealthy habits, in large part due to parents not having the time, energy, or resources for healthier home-cooked meals. Fast food establishments became the choice for my parents, who were also gaining weight and developing bad habits. Family meals became a scarcity and communication among the family diminished greatly. Additionally, the era of technology and increased screen time seems to promote everyone becoming more socially isolated and distant from both one another and their surroundings. Children are less and less physically active and often spend most of their time indoors on their phones, playing video games or watching Netflix or TV. My patients' mothers would frequently express to me their deep frustration and that they felt like failures because they could not provide as many home-cooked food, family activities, and quality time with their children as they wanted to. As these mothers confided in me about their frustration, I quietly acknowledged that I understood every word they said because that was exactly what I was experiencing and feeling. I, too, was a full-time working mother and feeling the heavy burden of both roles.

Many parents, both moms and dads, would tell me that their schedules were filled with so many mundane things to do each day. They yearned for simpler times when the family just did more spontaneous activities together, like when they were growing up. I slowly began to see more parents going on crash diets or getting gym membership at expensive health clubs to get back on track, but these plans inevitably failed. Today's parents are being tugged in all directions and end up paying little to no attention to their own health.

Social media nowadays offers answers to any of our questions at a click of a button. Some of it may be true, but a lot of the information is also misleading. Parents, as well as my teen patients, frequently ask me about the latest trends of popular diets or workouts to get their health back on track. In reality, I tell everyone that none of these quick fixes will ever work and if they did, I would hear about these amazing breakthroughs in my medical journals. In today's world of instant gratification, we seem more and more willing to throw our money away at quick fixes, but in reality, we simply end up where we started, gaining all, and even some extra, weight back.

As my practice grew over the years, I became acutely aware of how prevalent this feeling of families losing control, gaining more weight, and becoming unhealthier was. It was an unspoken, quiet desperation of hopelessness, and it felt like everyone in the family was destined for deteriorating health and family disconnectedness.

MY OWN STRUGGLES

As a full-time working mother of four young children in a similar situation, I was living these same challenges and frustrations in my own family. After being in private practice for a few years, it became difficult to take any time off or vacation time from my six-day workweek. We had a mortgage, private school tuition, preschool, daycare, and, of course, sustaining all the costs that go with operating our new private practices. In fact, after having my last two children, I returned to work within days after giving birth. Life then was not easy, and sometimes, you just do what you have to do.

I truly knew what my working moms were feeling, and my heart ached for all the families struggling with this dilemma of two working parents trying their best to get things in order. Previous generations of parents never had to face these issues because the majority of mothers stayed at home. I wanted families to be harmonious and happy again, even with two working parents. They, too, deserved that daily family time and connectedness. Somehow, I wanted to show others, as well as myself, that this could be done in a simple manner. Thus, this was the start of my new journey of figuring out ways to unite my family, as well as other families, and have them become stronger, happier, and healthier.

I truly believe that the answer to accomplishing this goal is getting everyone in the family to understand why it is so urgent to work together, as well as the many rewards they will reap once they embark on this life changing process. After conducting workshop sessions for families with obese and overweight children for many years, I could see that not only would parents enjoy a multitude of benefits from leading healthier lifestyles, but the children and the grandparents would also experience positive changes if they were all in with the program from the start.

THE IMPORTANCE OF THE FAMILY UNIT

This idea of involving the entire family is the secret ingredient of this revolutionary program and what has made me excited to share this solution I stumbled upon. It seemed to be working in our home, and I knew it could help the other families I was seeing on a daily basis who were in similar situations. Of course, the process of making lifetime changes would require commitment, time, patience, and lots of persistence from all family members. This is not a quick-fix plan, but I guarantee it will help to restore fun, laughter, better health, and unity to you and your family. Now, wouldn't you want to be a part of this program?

As a pediatrician, I began to witness how important the family unit was for the basic well-being of both parents and children. The family is the single most important influence in a child's life and those childhood years are crucial for their development. They need to feel the love and security of the family as well as have a sense of belonging.

I am always amazed that anyone can become a parent with no real training or preparation. We, as parents, strive to do our best, but in reality, we are probably just imitating what we remember our parents doing. However, most of our mothers of the previous generation did not have the stress of working a full-time job outside the home. Somehow, it seems imperative that a new model or shift in thinking of shared responsibility in the home evolves. Now, more than ever, the traditional roles of moms and dads need to be redefined. What's more, this may not be enough in the modern-day bustle. Engaging children, preferably at a young age, to contribute to the family each day is another key ingredient of healthy living and family harmony.

As I continued to work within my own family, as well as other families in my practice, I could see that things could definitely improve with just a few simple changes and some patience. This simple program is a proven way to reap enormous benefits of better health for the entire household through small modifications – and it is tailored to overcome your hectic schedules. The family unit can once again be strengthened, and everyone will be eager to return in the evening to the oasis of their home. That is my hope for you, dear reader, and the reason I'm writing this book. I promise you: help is within your reach.

I hope that my experience and expertise as a pediatrician and mother can help you start on a simple proven plan to better physical and emotional health, not only for you and your husband, but also for your children and your parents as well. As the many benefits start to unfold, you will clearly see that there is a light at the end of the tunnel, and it is never too late to start.

The tips, tricks, and secrets I have woven throughout this book are proven to be effective and can change your life and your family's life now. So, put on your seat belts, and let's get started on this journey today.

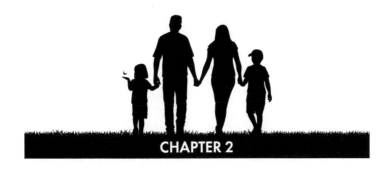

CHAPTER 2

WORKING PARENTS NEED HELP NOW – I GET IT

While growing up in the sixties and seventies, I began to witness a slow, evolving acceptance of women entering not only medicine but also engineering, business, and other male-dominated occupations. However, there were still many who did not believe that women belonged in these fields. I distinctly recall going to my assigned premed advisor as a freshman at the University of Hawaii, Manoa. The first words out of her mouth were, "I don't think you should go into medicine, and you need to consider another field of interest." I immediately grabbed my papers and never went back to her again.

In just three years, I went on to get my Bachelor of Science degree in biology with highest honors. Additionally, at the tender age of twenty, I gained early acceptance into the University of Hawaii John A. Burns School of Medicine at the start of my third year in college. I do sometimes wonder what would have happened if I took that premed advisor's advice, but I had my family's support and that was what mattered to me at the time. Just having one or two people in your corner believing in you can totally make the biggest difference.

My four years as a medical student were not easy and required many, many hours of study, but as a class, we bonded and worked together to help each other get through. By process of elimination, I decided that pediatrics would be my specialty.

MEETING AND MARRYING MY "BEST" FRIEND

During my freshman undergraduate year at the University of Hawaii, I was very blessed to make a new friend, Stephen Wee, who was also a premed student. We both hit it off, and he and I were in that "friend zone" for the next seven years. Most of all, he lived close by and always gave me rides in his cute light-blue Volkswagen Bug. You could say it was a relationship of convenience. He was such a great guy, and I never understood why he never had a girlfriend.

Finally, after seven years of brotherly friendship and free car rides, in our fourth and final year of medical school, he looked at me one evening we were out and said, "I think we should go for it" to which I replied, "Go for what? Ice cream?" After a few minutes of awkward silence, I finally realized that this was his marriage proposal, and he was asking me to marry him. I was caught so off guard, but as corny as this sounds, I realized what a genuinely wonderful man he was and knew I had to be with him for the rest of my life. And anyway, I still needed rides and all the many thoughtful things he always did for me without any complaints. I thought to myself, "Wow, I think I just won the lottery!"

So, I accepted this unique marriage proposal, and then we started to really date. We were married on May 24, 1980, in Honolulu, Hawaii, and off we went to Columbus, Ohio, for our respective residencies. I spent three years as a pediatric resident at Columbus Children's Hospital, now known as Nationwide Children's Hospital, and then went on to do an ambulatory fellowship there. This was followed by two years of finally having my first real job working in a private practice in the Westerville, Ohio, area, where I gained even more experience as a young primary care pediatrician. Stephen did his three-year internal medicine residency at Riverside Methodist Hospital and then went on to work for three years at the Lancaster, Ohio, emergency room.

THE SCARY REALITY OF HAVING YOUR OWN CHILD

We had our first of four children – what an eye-opener that was for both of us. My husband, an internal medicine specialist, and myself, a trained pediatrician, brought this little bundle of joy home. That first night home, I remember calling my mom in Hawaii and just crying over the phone, saying that I was a scared, inexperienced first-time parent and asking her to catch the next plane over to Ohio to help me. As I look back, this seems silly, especially as a trained pediatrician, but at the time, the feeling of responsibility and dependence of this baby on me was just so overwhelming. I tell many of the families I work with that I know exactly that feeling of fear and shock on their first night home with their newborn baby. As I have said many times before, I feel that my experience raising four children has been just as valuable as my pediatric residency training.

Four Children, Full-Time Doc, and the Slow Burnout

In 1984, with our second son on the way, we decided it was time to return to Hawaii. There was a new housing development coming up in Central Oahu. Despite the fact that this was away from the city and considered "country," we decided to buy a home there because just a few blocks up the road, there was a new vacant medical office building. We were the first tenants to lease a space there, and in 1984, we put up our signs and officially started our combined pediatric and internal medicine practices. It took nearly four years to build our private practices, so for those first few years, we both worked at other part time jobs as physicians to keep the lights on, pay for daycare, preschool, the home mortgage, and everything else.

We seemed to have such an idyllic life, with four healthy, active children, two growing medical practices, somewhat flexible hours, and a nice home. But underneath this façade, I was slowly getting smothered. I worked six days a week seeing patients in the office and then took my work home to finish up charting and making phone calls. I was on call twenty-four hours a day, 365 days a year to take care of emergencies. I made many trips commuting to the city to see, admit, and care for my critically ill patients at the Kapiolani Children's Hospital. This job of a pediatrician, caring for other people's children, left me with no energy for my own children and my husband at the end of the day. I didn't know it at the time, but I was slowly burning out. I kept saying to myself, *I am a professional woman*, and *I made it this far. I am capable of doing a great job as a full-time pediatrician and also as a full-time mom at home.*

The Breaking Point at Age Forty

At the age of forty, with four very active children all under the age of twelve, I began to experience a gradual decrease in my appetite, difficulty falling and staying asleep, loss of joy in most everything, and a feeling of an extremely heavy burden on my shoulders, daily. I felt this way for over a year and just barely made it from day to day. My husband and I, both physicians, could not figure out what was wrong with me. I cried often, felt hopeless, and yearned for the day when I could feel myself again.

The daily tasks of a mom working outside the home as well as keeping up with all the tasks of a mother of four children continued, despite what I was feeling, and I had to keep my happy face on. One day while reading a medical journal, I came across an article on the major signs of depression, and I finally self-diagnosed myself as being depressed. Within a week, I sought the care of a wonderful psychiatrist who immediately diagnosed me with depression and placed me on two weeks of leave from the office, antidepressants, and weekly therapy. Within weeks, I slowly crawled out of that dark hole and started to feel like myself once again. I was so relieved to finally see the light at the end of the tunnel.

At this point in my life, this episode of depression was a life changing wake-up call for me. I realized that I was not superwoman and could not do everything by myself. I needed to put my pride aside and humbly accept the help and support of my husband, children, parents, and in-laws. We sat down with everyone, including the children, and explained to them what was going on with *Mom*. We discussed the importance of everyone contributing to the family and making contributions based on their age and abilities. My husband also pitched in and helped even more in household chores. My parents and mother-in-law also helped with home-cooked meals, cleaning, occasional childcare, grocery shopping, and more.

Sometimes, the darkest parts in our lives can be the best places to learn. I gained so much insight into how overwhelmed a person can get and that at certain seasons in our lives, we have to accept help graciously and humbly. It was also a tough learning experience for me, but I truly believe this has made me a better mother and a more compassionate doctor. I could really relate to my working parents and the trials they were going through daily. Overall, I would not want to go through this again, but the lessons I learned from this challenging situation have stayed with me for life and enrich my life even more.

THE BANNER YEAR OF 2010

2010 was a banner year for me. My husband and I celebrated our thirtieth wedding anniversary with a two-week trip to China. This was the first time we took an overseas trip, and it was such a memorable, well deserved vacation. We were able to reminisce on the last thirty years of hard work and look forward to the next thirty years of married bliss and time together as empty nesters. The three older boys had graduated from college and the youngest, our daughter, had just turned twenty-one years old and was moving on to her final year at Westmont College in Santa Barbara. However, God had other plans in store for us.

On Friday, June 11, 2010, my husband, best friend, and business partner, died suddenly and unexpectedly in my arms, within minutes. We had just returned from our memorable vacation two weeks earlier and after seeing our morning patients, my husband told me he did not feel well. I did not think anything about this comment and immediately told him that I would heat up our lunches and be back. A few minutes later, when I returned with our lunches, he was dead.

He was only fifty-five years old and up until then, he had no known medical problems. In fact, he had just seen his primary care physician and had a clean bill of health. According to the autopsy report, he had an aortic aneurysm that ruptured. For the first few weeks, I went into utter shock and disbelief. I was numb, mad, sad, confused, and experiencing all kinds of emotions at once. In addition to all of this, I was informed by the real estate management company that my office lease was up in two weeks and they were going to more than double my rent and require me to sign the lease for no less than five or ten years. I declined to sign on these terms, so they gave me one year to vacate.

MY ANSWER FROM GOD

At this point in my life, I could have quit medicine and retired completely, which my four grown children vigorously encouraged me to do. However, there was something inside of me that kept saying it was not my time to quit medicine at the age of fifty-four years. I continued seeing my patients in the office and several of my husband's colleagues continued to graciously help out and see his patients as well. My practice was slowly going bankrupt, and I knew I had to vacate my office in a year. Things did not look good at all, in fact, they looked hopeless. My world had turned upside down, and it felt as if someone had ripped half of my heart out. My husband was the one and only real boyfriend I had, and now I was alone. Who am I? What is my purpose in life now? I had so many things to sort out. In the meantime, I had stopped attending church and felt so much anger toward God for taking my husband and business partner at such a young age.

One night, three months after my husband's sudden death, I went down on my knees and desperately cried out to God: "Please show me a sign about what you want me to do!" I waited for an answer and within five days, I got a call from someone referred to me by another physician stating that she had twenty years of experience as an office practice manager. She asked to meet with me and offered to help me out with my business. Could this be the sign from God I so desperately needed?

When she arrived, she told me I looked so distraught that she felt compelled to offer her services for free, until I could get back on my feet again to pay her. She looked me in my eyes and told me that she could turn my practice around, but before we went any further, she requested permission to pray for me. The only thought that came into my mind when she said this was this was certainly the sign from God that I requested a few days ago.

She started work immediately in my office and made the necessary changes for my new practice to make a turn-around. We renamed my practice "Wee Pediatrics, Inc." and began the hard work of rebuilding it. I was very blessed to find a brand-new empty office space up the road for sale, and it was double the size of my previous office. I decided to buy it and only through the grace of God, the loans went through. I began designing, planning, and constructing my new office.

In December 2011, just eighteen months after the death of my husband, I moved into my newly constructed office, the Wee Wellness Center. This was the start of my new chapter in my life as a business owner and solo practitioner, and I knew God had more plans in store for me.

FULFILLING MY PASSION IN LIFE

About one month after working for me, my office manager turned to me and asked me a question that no one had ever asked me before: "What is your passion?" I immediately replied that my passion had always been to help other working mothers and their families stay healthy, prevent obesity, and strengthen that all important family unit. This, coincidentally, was also a deep personal passion of hers. She had three daughters, and as a single mother for most of her life, she needed to work two to three jobs to support them. She had concerns similar to other working mothers, about providing the best meals and parenting her children the best she could with the limited time she had. Thus, in 2011, my office manager and I began free in-office workshops for my families with obese and overweight children who were ready for change. The families that participated had to agree to have the entire family attend five two-hour Saturday afternoon sessions. It was run by myself, my office manager, my staff and a host of other volunteers, including an army recruiter for physical training exercises at the park. We did several cohorts for the next couple of years with very positive results. As my practice got busier, these workshops had to eventually be postponed due to time constraints. However, I knew many of families out there still needed help.

Walk with a Doc – Oahu

In February 2016, with the help of UHA Health Insurance and their CEO, Howard Lee, I launched a chapter of the nonprofit organization, Walk with a Doc – Oahu, where I could now reach out to my entire community for a free weekly walking event. I invited people of all ages, fitness levels, and insurances to come and walk with me in the Central Oahu Regional Park, near the tennis courts, on Saturday, from 8:00 to 9:00 a.m. for health, fellowship, and fun. This free weekly event started out modestly, but soon word began to spread in the community and we now have approximately thirty to forty walkers each week. I share a new health tip weekly and then we stretch, walk for forty-five minutes, and finally cool down, followed by water and fruit refreshments, generously donated by Stay Fit Physical Therapy.

Earlier this year, we were able to kick off a new chapter of Walk with a Future Doc at the Kakaako Waterfront Park every fourth Sunday from 9:00 to 10:00 a.m. This is put on by our enthusiastic University of Hawaii John

A. Burns School of Medicine (JABSOM) medical students and faculty who also see the value of what community involvement can do for everyone. We recently established two other monthly programs every second Saturday: Hike with a Doc, from May to September and Dance with a Doc at nearby Pas de Deux Dance Studio from October to April. The purpose of these programs is to reach out to the community and help everyone become more active together in different venues. I believe the social interactions and just knowing that you are not alone in this journey makes all the difference. Over the past four years, I have heard amazing testimonials and seen great physical and emotional results from my walkers. Nearly every week, someone will come up to me with tears telling me that this was just that little nudge they needed to embark on their journey toward better health. As my walkers become healthier, I have seen some of them move on to other activities such as playing pickle ball, traveling the world, or participating in half marathons. As a physician, Walk with a Doc has given me immense satisfaction in knowing that I made a little difference in someone's life. I also feel grateful to my walkers for keeping me accountable for my own health. There are many Saturdays when I just want to sleep in and not attend, but I know my walkers are expecting me. After attending the walk, I feel so exhilarated and ready for the weekend. As my son recently reminded me, "Hey, Mom, you cannot become obese because you are the Walk with a Doc leader."

In early 2019, I was fortunate enough to receive a grant from the Aloha Care Community Intervention Program Wai Wai Ola Program. As a result of this, I was able to restart my workshop sessions for families with obese or overweight children. I conducted three cohorts, with five to six families in each group and named my program the Hawaii Healthy Family Revolution. The final results of our intervention for the three family cohorts are in, and they show not only positive physical benefits, such as decreased weight, percent body fat, and waist circumference, but also, most remarkably, positive mental benefits, including improved emotional well-being and improved depression scores in most of our participants. Additionally, 100 percent of the families felt ready and able to use the information obtained in this program to help with planning and decision-making for improving their health as well as their children's health.

The Hawaii Healthy Family Revolution Gains National Recognition

On September 8, 2019, I had the honor of presenting my Hawaii Healthy Family Revolution Program nationally at the 2019 Patient Centered Medical Home Congress held in Boston, Massachusetts. It was a great honor to share this with other like-minded colleagues from all across our country. It was received very well, and I will be following up with national groups, such as the Center for Disease Control. I was recently invited to speak at the 2020 International Obesity Chronic Disease Conference (IOCDC) on July 6, 2020, in San Francisco. I am very excited to have this opportunity to present my family workshops on an international level as well.

We are currently making plans for the coming year to reach out to companies or groups interested in having this program available to their employees. Additionally, I would like to continue these workshops for families ready for change and possibly extend it to adults and seniors as well. In the near future, I would like to approach health insurance companies and have them help cover participation in innovative programs like this. Our families desperately need help now, especially our children. This would be an amazing win-win situation, not only for health insurance companies down the road, but also for saving the family unit and getting people of all ages healthier and keeping them that way.

I continue to see patients in my office on a limited basis, as I have hired another pediatrician, Dr. Jordan Arakawa, to assist me with the daily office visits. Additionally, I have the privilege of serving as Pediatric Program Director for the Queens Akoakoa Physician Organization to advocate for and support our local pediatricians in this fast-paced changing medical payment model.

For the past two years, I have also had the honor of doing a monthly television children's health tip for a local morning news program, *Take2*, on KHON 2. Additionally, I have been doing many other guest segments on radio shows such as HPR's the *Body Show with Dr. Kathy Kozak, Community Matters with Rick Hamada, The Good Life with Dr. Danny Yamashiro* and the *Kupunawiki* Radio Show, as well as presentations to various schools and community groups.

My goal in the coming years is to continue to think of innovative ways to get the people of Hawaii healthier. My hope and dream are for people to know that health is truly your greatest wealth and it is never too late to start on this journey.

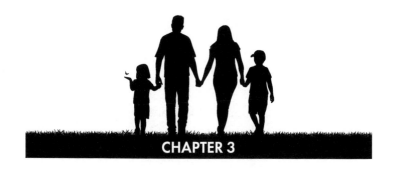

CHAPTER 3

THINKING OUTSIDE THE BOX IN TODAY'S WORLD

As a student of the sixties, my parents enrolled me in a very, at the time, popular speed-reading course called Evelyn Wood's Reading Dynamics. I'm not sure if I really know how to speed read, but the one takeaway that was extremely valuable for the rest of my life was to always preview or scan the book, front and back, looking at the table of contents and understanding what I wanted to get from reading the book.

In this chapter, I hope to give you an overview of the program so that you get an overall understanding of this unique approach toward better health for you and your entire family. The first and most important basis for success is the buy in and enthusiastic participation of all family members in the household. It is an all or nothing deal.

What I have found over the years is that if there is resistance by anyone, the family will have much more difficulty succeeding. If the majority of the family is on board, try to give the naysayer a gentle "nudge" and ask that person to at least give it a try. Once you get started, it is hard to stop, and soon the whole family is having a lot of fun. Another suggestion would be to discuss this with your primary care physician and see if he/she can give this family member a little "nudge" of encouragement.

The whole idea of this program is to encourage the entire family to develop healthy habits for a lifetime, so we certainly cannot leave a household member behind. I will give you basic information about nutrition and exercise in an easy-to-understand manner as well as tools your entire family can start to use right away toward achieving your goals.

Currently, there is so much information online about which new diets or exercises are the most effective that this information overload is so confusing for everyone, including physicians. The information I share with you on food and exercise will be simplified so that you will have a clear understanding when faced with the many choices out there.

MAKING CHANGES FOR A LIFETIME

In order for anyone to make lifestyle changes, it is important to make these changes gradually over time, so that it becomes a habit for life. Thus, a lot of valuable information will be presented, but my intent is for you and your family to sit down and make a joint decision, one small bit at a time. I will provide you with tools to use as a family, but you must choose the one simple change you and your family would like to start with.

MY PLATE AND 5210

You will learn basic nutritional information such as the valuable My Plate illustration as well as the 5210 concepts to help you become healthier immediately. I will also talk about one of the major causes of excessive weight gain in America today, which is sugar-sweetened beverages. Wherever you go nowadays, whether it is fast-food chains, restaurants, parties, or simply at home, the menus and our refrigerators are filled with these sugar-sweetened beverages. In fact, most places allow you to have unlimited amounts of these beverages or super-size it for the same price as a small. It has been my experience when teaching families in my workshop, that this topic is the number-one most popular, eye-opening take away lesson they learned.

FAMILY AWARENESS OF SLEEP AND BREAKFAST

Additionally, many other factors come into play when we are talking about controlling weight gain, low energy, and chronic fatigue. The two most important factors that will be discussed in detail are sleep and breakfast. These are two of the most important factors in helping one maintain a healthy weight and prevent the pounds from adding up over time. I will share ideas on different ways you and your family can be successful in attaining the adequate amount of sleep and making time for breakfast, both of which are always challenges for many families.

Since this is a family-based program, I will touch on the importance of getting children, of all ages, involved in the planning, prepping, and actual cooking of the meals. This gets everyone helping out and the kids can take pride and ownership in what they have helped prepare. This will lead to not only more family connectedness, but everyone will be more likely to eat the healthy meals they helped create.

One of the crucial steps in this program is understanding that screen time is a great robber of personal and family time. You will understand that the sooner you set boundaries and rules, as parents, on screen time, the more likely the children will comply. We call this a media plan, and this is a discussion that must be ongoing and adjusted based on the child's age and needs. It is also important that the parents or guardians also adhere to these guidelines so that the children can see the consistency being adhered to.

SETTING GOALS

The next important chapter is devoted to equipping you with tools for setting and achieving small goals as a family. For any habit to become a part of your routine, one needs to do it for thirty straight days. You will learn to use the S.M.A.R.T. approach, and each part of this approach is detailed and taught to you in an easy-to-understand manner.

Once the program swings into full action, it will be important for everyone in the household to keep each other accountable too, working toward the family goals. Additionally, I will discuss the importance of setting mealtimes, bedtimes, family routines, and schedules, and sticking to them consistently. By keeping everyone "on track," success as a family is inevitable with time and patience.

BE PRESENT IN THE MOMENT

There are two very valuable concepts that I introduce in the program and that is the important roles of mindfulness and meditation. The world as it is today is so busy, and everything is moving so quickly around us. However, in the rush to get our work done by multitasking, we may be losing touch with the present moment. We are missing out on what we are doing or what we are feeling. Mindfulness is the practice of purposely focusing your attention on the present moment and accepting it without any judgment. In many new studies coming out now, mindfulness appears to have many health benefits, including stress reduction and increasing overall happiness. I will teach basic mindfulness meditation and the popular method of doing this through focusing on your breathing or other bodily sensations.

BE GRATEFUL ALWAYS

Finally, we will discuss why practicing an attitude of gratitude is beneficial for everyone's well-being and success in life. Gratitude is about feeling and expressing appreciation for all that you have received. This is a skill to develop, and it can change your perspective on life. There is always something to be grateful for, no matter how many negative things keep coming at you. Gratitude helps us stop focusing on the day-to-day annoyances and instead lets us see more clearly the abundance in our lives. Study after study is coming out on the benefits of practicing and journaling gratitude in both our physical and emotional well-being as well as strengthening our relationships and encouraging us to pay it forward.

I have a plaque up on my office wall, and I try to live by this motto daily: "Live like it's your last day." I have learned that in life, there are no guarantees. Every day is a precious gift, and what we do with this gift is our choice. I hope your choice, like mine, will be to make every breath and day count.

MAINTAIN PROGRESS AND KEEP MOVING FORWARD

Finally, I will show ways you and your family can maintain ongoing progress and momentum forward to accomplish your goals. It is always easy to get excited and dive into a new program, but it is another story when it comes to keeping everyone engaged and participating. Again, as a reminder, this program is about a lifetime of change. Everyone must understand from the start that noticeable changes are not going to happen on day one or even the first week. Instead, time, patience, and consistency are needed in heavy doses for success.

As a family unit, it will be important to remind one another of the family goals and express "high fives" for a job well done. I will be talking about having weekly family talk time to discuss what is working and what is not working so that goals can be modified, if needed. It will be essential to be intentional on planning scheduled family activities throughout the week as well as the weekends. Also, at this time, the family can reflect on their progress and how far everyone has come since the start of the program. By being grateful for the accomplishments and hard work of the entire family, I highly encourage all my families to share this program with their relatives and friends. I will help you understand that by helping other families in similar situations, you will continue to reinforce your own success and continue to reap greater rewards as a family.

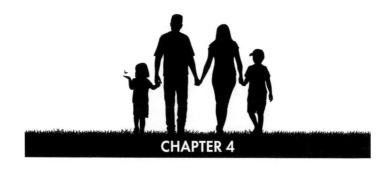

CHAPTER 4

FAMILY TEAMWORK IS THE KEY TO SUCCESS

While I was growing up, my maternal grandparents from China lived with us for many years. I remember feeling so embarrassed to have these old folks at our home and refused to have any of my friends come over. Family, for me, meant there were eight of us in one household: my maternal grandparents, mother, father, three siblings, and myself. There were always so many chores to do: meals to cook, clothes to wash, and other essential activities that had to be done daily. We even had our very own vegetable garden in our backyard, which was tenderly cared for by my grandfather. We also had a variety of fruit trees, which continually supplied us with fruits throughout the year. As a young girl, all I could think of was how weird our family seemed to be. I always wished I could have lived in a normal American household like *Leave It to Beaver*, which I saw on TV.

Little did I know then that living in this large household was such a blessing in disguise because it taught me many lessons that I used later with my own family. My mom rarely used our clothes washer and dryer and would instead prefer to wash clothes by hand. I was often assigned to hang the clothes on the line in our backyard and bring them in to fold, iron, and put away. We did have a dishwasher, but I cannot remember a single time it was ever used. I had no Fitbit or pedometer back then, but I always knew I had plenty of daily physical activity. We had one television in our entire home, and I remember looking forward to Sunday evenings, when we all gathered around it, including my grandfather, to watch Walt Disney's Wonderful World of Color followed by the TV show *Bonanza*.

As a multigenerational family living in the same home, we were constantly with each other, eating, prepping meals, doing chores, watching television, and, of course, fighting. As I look back now, life seemed so simple, and helping the family was a must. As children we never got allowances, but at the end of the day, it was nice to know that we each contributed to the family.

In today's world, technology and material possessions have overtaken us, and we are constantly using appliances such as the dishwashers, washing machines, dryers, robot vacuums, remote controls for the TV, and many more. Today, there is barely any need to get off our couches. No one has any time for gardening, so instead we go to supermarkets and get giant boxes of processed foods, smoothies, muffins, croissants, and other goodies. Once at home, everyone microwaves their own dinner and immediately goes into their own rooms to eat. We even text one another, even though we are all at home, and we rarely have any time for one-on-one conversation. We are supposed to be a family, but instead it feels like we are all only roommates living in the same house.

PARENTING TOGETHER CONSISTENTLY

Over the years, I have found that when the parents or guardians of the household can come together with clear ideas about goals or schedules and present them as a united front, the rest of the family will follow. A strong leadership team is essential for formulating which direction everyone will take. If there are disagreements or lack of communication between the parents or guardians, children will immediately pick up on this, even at a very young age. As parents, we each come from very different upbringings, values, and parenting styles. It is now essential to discuss and decide jointly with your partner on how you want to raise your children. The values and lessons we leave them will hopefully lead to a happy and fulfilling life. In most cases, once you have had these discussions, you each become clear about which direction you want to take. This process makes it so much easier to have the entire family on board with the plans.

You Can Choose Your Parenting Style

There were many things I loved about my childhood growing up, but then there were other things I felt could have been better. As a parent, I now had a second chance to do it over with my children. For example, when growing up, my parents never gave us a lot of physical hugs and kisses, but I always knew they loved me. As a young parent, I discussed with my husband that I wanted our children to learn that hugging and kissing was the norm, and we agreed we would practice this daily from the time they were born. As a result, we hugged and kissed each other in front of them and gave our children abundant physical affection, which continues to feel very natural for them. This is the beauty of parents talking to one another, not making any assumptions, and moving forward as a united pair.

REKINDLE THE ROMANCE

One of my favorite question to ask my families during the office visit is "When was the last time you went out on a date together, without the children?" I will even ask this question when their child is just one month old. It is so easy to get sucked up into the overwhelming daily activities that demand your attention when you have children, especially a newborn. I have seen how this soon leads to dads feeling left out and isolated. In some cases, some of the dads even get kicked out of their beds, and the child becomes the center of the entire family. As parents and the leaders of the family, it is so important to communicate and understand each other's struggles, frustrations, and feelings. The family unit has the parents at the head and the children secondary. You have to have these separate date nights or quiet times together to rekindle and recharge your bond as parents, which will help you see your roles more clearly. Once this is established, it makes parenting so much easier when you work as a team and understand who is in charge.

The children also benefit greatly, as they see their parents spending quality time together and have the opportunity to see what a successful marriage actually looks like. I do believe that this is a wonderful legacy to leave children and they will, in turn, mimic it in their own lives as adults.

Once this hierarchy is established, where parents are the heads of the family, the schedules, routines, and other family activities become so much easier to enforce. The children know that there are certain boundaries that cannot be crossed and also know where their position is in the family.

For myself and my husband, we decided early on in our marriage that we would have "sacred" Saturday date nights. Just the thought of a date with my husband without children at the end of the week made my entire work week bearable. It was pretty simple: dinner at our favorite Chinese restaurant, followed by going to the $1.00 movie theater. These quiet times we had together were priceless and really helped us connect on a much deeper level as husband and wife. I really appreciated this time to recharge every weekend to be fully present with my husband and plan for our future.

THE CRUCIAL QUESTION FOR THE DAY

As our four children were growing up, my husband and I always had one question we asked them every evening.

That question was, "What did you do for the family to-day?" When we came home from work, we could often hear the children scurrying around frantically putting their shoes in order, emptying the rubbish, cleaning their rooms, and so on, just so they could give us a good report. As two working parents, we had to involve the children in the household chores early on. We would always tell them that if we could finish the chores in time, then we could all go out and have time to do something fun. Looking back, some of these free family activities were the best memories we can recall. They were activities like riding bicycles, all six of us, around our little community, going to the park, or just playing outside with the neighborhood kids.

Let's Talk about the Day

Back in the days when we were on a strict budget, my husband and I decided not to pay for cable or have an Xbox in our home. If I recall correctly, we were the last holdouts for this on our street, and our poor boys were forced to visit the neighbors to get their fill of cable TV or video games. At one point, one of our sons even looked me in the eye and asked, "Why can't we be a normal family?" To which I immediately told him that we were the most normal family on our block, he just did not know it yet. There were many times when my husband and I wondered if we were being too strict, but you just keep moving forward and do the best you can with what you have.

One of the best things we ever did as a family was gathering together every evening to talk about the day before going to sleep. It was a family ritual that we kept going, even when the kids were in high school. We would all come together at about 8:00 p.m., after we read them books and everyone did their nighttime rituals. There, each person would have to say one thing that stood out about their day. It could be anything, and if anyone refused to contribute, they had to sit on the dreaded staircase landing "halfway up and halfway down." It was a nice time of reflection on that particular day and made all of us pause together to reflect. Most of all, it kept us informed about each other and as I look back, it bonded us tightly as a family. It forced us to practice our communication skills and at times even made it easier to address more difficult topics later on. During these nighttime talks as a family; we would take this opportunity to make special announcements of any major changes coming up or other important schedule changes. If my husband and I wanted input from the children, we would ask for their opinions, but they always knew that my husband and I would only take their ideas under advisement, as my husband and I would have the final say.

BE KIND TO THE PEOPLE YOU LOVE

Family members are the people you love the most, but with that being said, you sometimes forget your manners and occasionally do not speak to them in a loving manner. This was something I really had to work on often at home. After listening to crying and screaming children all day as a pediatrician, I would come home to my four young, active children and only see the total chaos the house was in. Before I could even put my briefcase down, all four children would be running to me and craving for my individual attention. I would have a thousand things in my head to do and just start shouting out to them what had not yet been done. There came a point where I felt that no one heard or saw me, as if I was invisible. When Dad came home later, he was greeted much more warmly, as he sat down and looked them in the face and listened to them. Finally, after much observation, I realized I needed to simply put my briefcase down, spend those first five minutes talking to the kids, who had missed me all day, and explain to them what the plans were for the next hour and my expectations for them. At the same time, I had to deliberately be aware of how I was speaking to or treating them, just as I would with my patients and their parents all day. I found that by simply being kinder and acting more loving, I had much more success in getting their cooperation. Kids just want to know that you love them.

I learned the hard way that our children just want to know that we care for them, and if we gave them even five minutes of undivided attention, they would be happy and satisfied. When they were younger, we had an annual tradition each Easter, where we would have an Easter egg hunt in our backyard. The eggs each had little presents like candy, coins, or promissory notes of five or ten minutes with Mom or Dad.

One Easter, I overheard the kids trying to trade their candies or coins for the notes that promised five or ten minutes with Mom or Dad and immediately saw that they actually cherished the time they had with us more than material things.

EVERYONE BENEFITS FROM FAMILY CONNECTEDNESS

As we continue to move forward in life as a family, whenever we want to make alterations or corrections along the path of life, it is crucial to set up the family as the main unit and have the parents be the definitive leaders. The alignment of the adults in charge makes it so much easier for everyone in the family to follow along without any hesitation. This process should begin when the children are infants, but it is never too late to start. As families succeed in getting the buy-in of the children, this same type of behavior follows the children in daycare and school. The respect, obedience, and teamwork the children have learned in the home become a pattern for them outside the home. They know their place and their boundaries and will comply with the instructions given to them. Life becomes so much easier for them at home and in school, and the rewards of working together as a team become a habit for a lifetime. As parents, one of the greatest gifts we can bestow on our children is that they are valued in a loving family. Teach them self-control and respect for others. Model a devoted marriage so that they choose their own partners based on this ingrained knowledge. This is how they grow strong enough to take on the challenges of adult life.

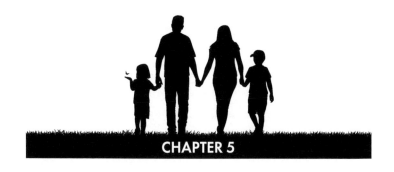

CHAPTER 5

NOURISHING OUR BODIES DAILY

LIFE IS FULL OF DECISIONS

There is no way around this fact – we all need to eat and nourish our bodies daily. We are making decisions all day long about what to eat, when to eat, and how much we are going to put in our mouths. This may be a conscious or an unconscious decision resulting from decades of learning.

From my early childhood, I recall many memories of going into the backyard and picking the vegetables we were going to have for dinner in the evening. We would have green beans, bitter melon, squash, and various herbs like green onions. For fruits, we would pick whatever was in season for that month and have that over and over till it was all gone from the tree.

In our modern world of fast-paced busyness, we no longer have this luxury. When my children were growing up, it was off to the nearby Costco to do our weekly run for the week. Having four hungry mouths to feed always presented a challenge, especially when they came along for the shopping experience. I recall grabbing those twelve-pack muffins or croissants and maybe even a large tub of ice cream or chips to satisfy their unending appetites. Of course, we would also make sure to get the bread, milk, fruits, and meats for the rest of the meals, but some of those other treats were so inexpensive that you just could not resist it for the price.

Currently, in our media-savvy world, there is so much information out there about what you should or should not eat. It is even confusing for physicians to keep up with the latest research. I remember many years ago, when I was growing up, we were told to eat margarine instead of but-ter, but now it is known that there are too many trans fats in margarine and we should go back to butter. No wonder it is confusing to figure out what you can and cannot eat.

The one motto I have stuck with throughout the years of being a mom and pediatrician is that there is no such thing as a forbidden food. Every food has its place in mod-eration. As a first-time mom, I know I was very strict with my firstborn son. With good intentions, I tried my best to keep candies and other sweets away from him when he was a young child. However, as he got older and entered school, this strategy backfired on me. I caught him with a lot of candy wrappers under his bed, and I found out this had been going on for a while. With the rest of the three children, I took a different and more relaxed approach, which turned out much better. They were allowed sweets, but always in moderation. Whenever there were special occasions or holidays, like Christmas or Halloween, they were able to have their treats, just not on a daily basis.

MY PLATE

Many years ago, we all followed the famous "Food Pyramid" recommendations for healthy eating. The older food pyramid was introduced in 1991 and was supposed to be our nutrition guide for everyone. However, in reality, it was confusing and not helpful in meal planning for the general population. In May 2011, this Food Pyramid was ditched and replaced by the new My Plate.

The major difference between these two models was less emphasis on grains. The MyPlate version reserves only one fourth quadrant for whole grains, one fourth quadrant for protein and the remaining half of the plate focuses on vegetables and fruits. The My Plate model does not mention how many servings you should eat of any particular food group. Assuming you are eating off a normal-size nine-inch plate and if you don't pile your food too high, then you are probably eating a normal, healthy amount of food for good weight management. This at least gives you a framework and goal to work toward. It also makes you aware of the importance of fruit and vegetable intake.

Since we must all eat daily, it is important to understand that we must try our best to get all the required nutrients, both macronutrients and micronutrients, for great health. Our foods can be further analyzed and classified based on their composition. Food labels now help us break down these foods and list the macronutrients and micronutrients so that we know exactly what we are about to consume. First, macronutrients provide us with calories, or energy that our bodies need to make it through the day. They are separated into three categories: carbohydrates (four calories per gram), fats (nine calories per gram), and finally proteins (four calories per gram). Second, micronutrients are the substances we eat in trace amounts that our bodies require to function; unlike the macronutrients, they do not give us any energy. Micronutrients are commonly known as vitamins and minerals that foods can provide. Various health conditions as well as certain diets can lead to deficiencies in micronutrients.

THE DILEMMA OF PICKY EATERS

Many of the families I work with frequently tell me that their children hate vegetables. They have tried a certain vegetable two or three times and each time their child refused it. However, I emphasize the "try a bite rule," where a certain food must sometimes be tried seven to ten times before a child actually likes it. I have seen this work in my patients as well as my own children. It is also important to note that parents and other adults should be good role models and also go along with this rule. I tell parents to allow the child to use all their senses when trying something new. For example, they can use their fingers to feel its texture, their nose to smell it, their lips and tongue to take a small taste of it and finally a small bite with their teeth. If they want to spit it out, they have that right, but not in a big dramatic way. Their efforts to try a new food or one they think they dislike should be acknowledged, not praised in a grandiose manner, before moving on.

Another very valuable concept I tell parents to put up in their kitchen is the following rule:

Parents Decide:

- What food is served; and
- When the food is served

Children Decide:

- Whether or not to eat; and
- How much to eat

By remembering this, it will make mealtimes so much simpler. Both the parents and children are clear on what is expected at mealtime. No more shouting, scolding, or negotiating – it is what it is, and this is how it is always going to be. Believe it or not, this rule will actually help get picky eaters eating better. Try it!

THE TAKE IT OR LEAVE IT RULE

When our four children were growing up, I had a sign I found that read, "You have two choices for your meal today, 'Take it or leave it.'" I grew up with this rule, and I was determined not to be a short order chef, making separate meals for each family member and my children knew it. If one of them chose not to eat, they could excuse themselves, but they were not allowed to have their meal reheated or any additional snacks or milk. They could only have water until the next meal/snack. If that meant going to sleep hungry, then so be it, but I tell the families I work with that in all my years of practice, I have not lost a single child to starvation after skipping one meal or snack. Once the children understand the rules, they will realize the need to eat what is presented in front of them. Thus, the benefit of being firm and consistent in this manner teaches your children, especially when they are at a young age, to eat what everyone else is eating, and, in the end, they will grow up to be great eaters as adults. In essence this is the solution to a picky eater, but if it is not done early on, you are going to get a lot of pushback. Once again, the entire family, including the family caretakers, must all be on board with this rule, or it will not work.

A final note on offering praise to children when they do eat their meal or snack. Be careful about offering an excessive amount of praise simply for eating their meals. Your children will see your response and feel more inclined to continue eating, despite feeling satisfied, to please you. Over the years, I have seen this strategy backfire and many of these children go on to become overweight or obese adults. They continue to overeat, as this is what was learned in childhood, and habits, whether good or bad, are always difficult to break.

5210 MANTRA

The second important concept I want to discuss is called the 5210 rule. This is a compilation of many rules for what contributes to a healthy lifestyle that health experts world-wide created. After much discussion and debate, it was narrowed down to the following:

- five servings of vegetables, roots, or fruits a day
- two hours or less of screen time
- one hour of physical activity daily
- zero sugar-sweetened beverages daily

This easy-to-understand concept has been adapted across our nation, and it is applicable to all ages. In Hawaii, we have adopted this program and have called it the Hawaii 5210, Let's Go Program. As a member of the Hawaii 5210 Board, I have tried over the years to get this message out to our entire state, including our outer islands. We have distributed posters and flyers in schools, after-school programs, YMCAs, YWCAs, sports programs, physician offices, community colleges, and any other program that touches our youth. The goal is to present a unified message of what constitutes good health over our entire state and help our families address healthy living in a simplified manner. If everyone can learn, understand, and make changes, whenever possible, then these 5210 programs will achieve its purpose.

When looking at the 5210 information, one of the questions that always comes up during our workshop sessions is "what is a serving size?" Of course, for very young children, their plates should be smaller, and servings should be given according to their size. However, for the majority of us, the following guidelines will also help:

- one serving of vegetables: one cup of raw vegetables or half a cup of cooked vegetables.
- one serving of fruit: half a cup of cut-up fruits or one medium-size fruit, about the size of a tennis ball
- one serving of meat protein: two palm-size servings per day
- one serving of a snack: one handful of nuts or small candies or two handfuls for chips or pretzels

THE HAZARDS OF SUGAR-SWEETENED BEVERAGES

The one topic that is of crucial importance when it comes to what is contributing to the obesity crisis today is the ever-presence of sugar-sweetened beverages. The 5210 rules state that zero to very little sugar-sweetened beverages should be consumed. As a shopper, I see so many families buying gallons of fruit punch, 100 percent orange juice, or crates of sodas, Gatorade, sweetened iced tea, Capri Sun packets, and energy drinks. For many years, we always thought fresh-squeezed orange or apple juice was healthy. The reality is that one cup of concentrated fruit juice has a high concentration of sugar that is similar to the amount of sugar in a can of soda. One cup of orange juice contains the sugar level of five to six oranges, and drinking one or two cups of this will give you an extremely large amount of sugar in just a few minutes' time. Now, contrast this to eating five oranges in one sitting, which is virtually impossible to do. First, it would take too long to peel them and then eating five whole oranges would fill you up due to all the healthy fiber. My advice has always been to save your money and eat whole fruits instead of buying juices. If you really love 100 percent juices, then by all means go ahead and serve this occasionally, but no more than half a cup or four ounces a day. Another trick is to dilute half of your cup of juice with water.

Again, the habits and tastes we are developing in our children, as well as ourselves, will gradually take hold. After cutting back on sugar-sweetened beverages, you will find that they are too sweet, and water or milk will be your fluids of choice. I encourage everyone to be knowledgeable of the drinks they have daily as just these sugar-sweetened beverages alone can lead to a lifetime of steady weight gain. I personally have nothing against having one or two of this type of drink on the weekend or for special occasions. We just need to know that we cannot have these daily and always think "moderation."

Recently, at one of my family workshops, a dad lost five pounds in five weeks just by eliminating the one or two sodas he was drinking daily. If you can eliminate one soda can a day, it is predicted that you will lose a total of fifteen pounds a year if you do nothing else. Now that is something to think about.

Be cautious with artificial sweeteners. There have been studies showing that people who often drink artificially sweetened drinks, such as diet sodas, actually end up gaining more weight than those who do not use these. The reason for this is that artificial sweeteners trick our brains into thinking we are hungry, thus causing us to eat more throughout the day. Once again, I am reminded of my initial motto of moderation in your eating and drinking habits. When I go out for dinner on the weekends, I love a weekly can of soda or orange juice; I feel I can reward myself for being so good throughout the entire week. For me, this satisfies my cravings, and I look forward to having a sugar-sweetened beverage the following weekend.

A WORD ON SMOOTHIES

Smoothies have gained a lot of popularity recently, and many of the families I work with are doing these more and more. There are some families that even have smoothies daily for their morning meals. The trouble with smoothies is that you are getting more calories and sugar when you drink a smoothie rather than eating whole fruits or vegetables. Even if you make a smoothie at home, using only fruits and vegetables, you can drink it in a few minutes, compared with the fifteen or twenty minutes it would take to eat the same amount of fruits and vegetables whole. And if you're drinking smoothies frequently, you are probably consuming a lot more fruits than you would otherwise.

Even though smoothies do contain fiber, this fiber has been pulverized in the blending process and has turned the fruit into a thick paste. Thus, you are losing out on the fiber and its benefit. Fiber comes from plants and cannot be broken down or absorbed by your digestive tract. It not only keeps you regular but also helps lower cholesterol, keeps your blood sugar stable, makes it easier to lose weight, and may even keep you alive longer. As a result of pulverizing the fiber in the fruits and vegetables in your smoothie, you are likely to feel hungrier soon after drinking it than you would have if you had eaten the same amount of fruits and vegetables alone.

For children, I feel it is extremely important for them to learn, early on, what each individual fruit or vegetable tastes, smells, and feels like, rather than simply blending it into one drink. Also, beware of smoothies that are commercially made or store-bought, as they often contain added sugar, honey, or other sweeteners. There is a fine line between a smoothie and a milkshake. Remember, just because there is a leafy green in it does not make it low-calorie. The bottom line is you want to use smoothies as a way to boost nutrition but avoid using them or overusing them as a meal by themselves.

IMPORTANCE OF WATER AND MILK

So, what can you drink? There are two fluids for all age: water and milk. Calcium is an extremely important part of your daily diet, for all ages. Cow's milk would be the first choice, as one cup of milk has approximately 300 milligrams of calcium per eight-ounce cup. As the children grow and get into those crucial growing teen years, it is recommended that they have about 1,000 to 1,200 milligrams of calcium a day in addition to water. Studies show that today less than 15 percent of our teens are getting adequate calcium daily. Additionally, I remind parents that we, as adults, should also be drinking milk and getting our daily calcium of approximately 1,000 milligrams a day or about two to three cups to prevent osteoporosis and maintain our current bone mass. Once again, it is vital for the adults in the house to be good role models.

My current recommendation is to drink skim milk, which has zero percent fat, for everyone two years and older. For children one to two years of age, regular whole milk is advised, as the extra fat is necessary for critical brain growth.

Another interesting fact I want to share with you when deciding which cow's milk to buy is the following:

- one cup of whole milk (3 percent fat) is equal to the fat of eight strips of bacon
- one cup of 2 percent milk is equal to the fat of four strips of bacon
- one cup of 1 percent milk is equal to the fat of two strips of bacon
- 1 cup of skim milk is equal to zero fat

Currently, cow's milk is the preferred choice of milk. If you are lactose intolerant, you can choose plant-based milks. Currently, studies are still pending on plant-based milks as some of these may not have all the nutrients of regular cow milk. This is where reading labels is essential to understand what you are getting before buying.

READING FOOD LABELS

Learning how to read food labels is an important skill when shopping. Whenever looking at food labels, it is important to first scan the serving size. For example, one twenty-four-ounce can of Arizona Green Tea has about thirteen table-spoons of sugar, and if you read the food label carefully, you will see that this one can consists of three serving sizes. Thus, one serving of this beverage would make up just eight ounces (one cup) or one-third of the contents of the entire can. If you are like most people who drink this beverage, you drink the entire can in one sitting.

Another good label reading practice is searching for the sugar content in breakfast cereals. Always look at the serving sizes and then the sugar content. Generally, if a cereal has over fourteen grams of sugar per serving, then it is probably too sweet. Through my workshops, many of the families I work with, including the children, learn to become label readers and more informed consumers. I encourage families to shop together and really examine food labels to get the best value. This can be a game changer in improving overall health choices. For myself, I used to buy many preprocessed ready-to-eat frozen foods in bulk, but after reading food labels and seeing the amount of fat and sodium in these foods, it has changed my buying habits.

It is always best to stay with simple whole foods and assembling the food together in your kitchen on your own, without all the added preservatives and chemicals.

My final piece of advice is to try to choose foods that are lower in fat, cholesterol, sodium, and sugar. Instead, look for foods higher in fiber and any of the vitamins, minerals, and protein. As we discussed earlier in this chapter, those micronutrients (vitamins and minerals) and fiber are essential every day for proper bodily functions. Your body will thank you for your wiser choices.

MEAL PREP AS A FAMILY

Sit down as a family and talk about the food choices that are available. Check out the weekly food ad specials and buy what is in season or on sale. Based on this, plan your menu around these foods and take the entire family to shop with your list. Sometimes, shopping at the farmers' market can be more affordable since it goes from farm to table, so check that out on the weekends as a family activity. I also like Costco as an alternative to fresh fruits and vegetables, as it has a wide assortment fruits and vegetables in its freezer section. Many times, I also like the convenience of the small frozen Birdseye vegetable boxes that can be placed in the microwave and on the table in just a few minutes.

Get the children to wash and help prep the fruits and vegetables or participate in the cooking, if they are old enough. This gets everyone excited about the final product and more likely to eat the masterpiece they have helped to create.

Another great family idea is starting your very own vegetable garden at home. It could be as simple as getting a five-gallon plastic tub and planting a tomato plant or even herbs. The excitement of harvesting the first tomato, washing it, and then eating it is indescribable. The children become so connected to the earth, their plant, and the fruit of their labor, they become eager for more.

THINK OUTSIDE THE BOX

One of the questions I heard daily from my family was "What's for dinner, Mom?"

When feeding my family many years ago, I quickly discovered that everyone loved their meat. In fact, when my teenaged boys came home after school, I would have to label the container with meat with a large sign reading, "This is for dinner – do not eat this." Thus, there were many meals when I would serve everyone their portion of meat and the rest of the meal could be supplemented by other choices on the table. I always liked to have a green tossed salad available, along with brown rice, stir fry vegetables, and a frozen vegetable as well as a fruit served. Additionally, I loved to make large pots of hearty homemade soups to also offer as appetizers or serve with meals.

For breakfast, I did not limit our menu to just traditional "breakfast foods," but rather, I would pull out leftovers from the night before and offer more of these vegetables and fruits. If there were leftovers from breakfast, the remainder would be packed up for lunches. I continue to practice this daily with my own lunches. My staff teases me that I am the "Tupperware Queen" of portion control, and they always want to see the potpourri of food I'm having for my lunch. For me, the best part of my workday is my lunch.

I am not going to lie, but as a busy young mother, there were some days when I absolutely had to buy from fast-food establishments or takeout from restaurants. I would get your basic burgers, chicken tenders, pizza, or entrée and bring it home. I would then supplement this meal with lettuce salad, tomatoes, cheese, milk, water, and fruits. In Hawaii, we have something called plate lunches, and these would consist of a protein, two scoops of white rice, and macaroni salad. If I brought these plate lunches home, I would again supplement this meal with the fruits, veggies, water, and milk. One of my favorite ways to stretch a dinner meal was to go to Panda Express and pick up combo plates or the "Family Feast," and then take it home to add even more vegetables to the stir fry entrées. For example, I would stir fry fresh broccoli in the beef broccoli entrée, and many times, no additional seasoning was needed. Everyone would get their vegetables for dinner, but my kids always knew what I did and would roll their eyes.

For each family, figure out what works for you. Sit down as a family to discuss the many options for healthier choices that get everyone excited and start at this point. I guarantee it will slowly start to snowball into other exciting projects and great choices.

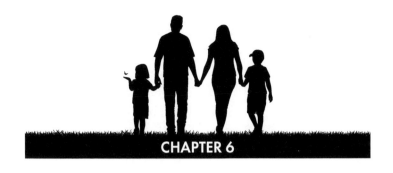

CHAPTER 6

JUST MOVE MORE

KIDS ARE NO LONGER "FREE RANGE"

Growing up in Hawaii, where the weather is sunny and eighty degrees year-round with only occasional light showers, it made it so easy to want to be outdoors all the time. Of course, those good old days were days of innocence – once we completed our household chores, our parents forced my siblings and me to play outside until it was dinner time. We had so much fun outdoors with the neighborhood kids playing with cardboard boxes, looking for earth worms, and just roller-skating up and down the street without a care in the world. I do not recall any twenty-four-hour fitness gyms, Curves, or any other exercise facilities back then. The only exercise class I ever saw as a child was the *Jack LaLanne Show* on the few television channels we had then. I remember following along and listening to his health tips. I especially loved seeing his lovely wife, Elaine, come in to help out.

For me, exercise was just moving around and something that I did daily, without even thinking about it. I did not have PE in elementary or middle school, but we always had recess and lunch, where I loved to play tetherball, volleyball, or just run around like a crazy person till sweat was streaming down the side of my face. Now that was a great workout!

Now let's fast-forward to today. As a mother of four young children, I frequently did not allow them to play outdoors by themselves. I remember reading a very popular book at the time named *Don't Talk to Strangers*. Back in the eighties, there was a young boy named Adam Walsh who was kidnapped from Sears and then found murdered. Many more horror stories kept coming up like Ted Bundy, the serial killer, and finally we had the tragedy of September 11, 2001. I remember it was Tuesday morning in Hawaii and our entire family just watched the live broadcast in disbelief as the second tower came falling down. Thus, in this new and modern changing world, my children were rarely allowed to be "free range" as I had so many things to do once I got home and did not have the time and energy to be outside supervising them. As they got older, it was always a struggle for more freedom, but again I always felt like I had to have a tight rein on them considering the world as it is today.

SELF-CARE TOSSED ASIDE

Caring for myself seemed like a luxury I could not afford while raising the kids and working full time. I had neither money nor time for a gym membership. In my younger, single days, I loved to jog, swim, or play tennis as much as possible. I considered work as my exercise when doing things like cleaning the kitchen, showers, and toilets; sweeping; cooking; grocery shopping; raking leaves; and all the other things mothers do. At the office, I was on my feet constantly, jumping from room to room to see my patients and frequently wrestling with patients to give them their shots. Throughout all of this, I felt very resentful for having to do it all and felt like I never had a good attitude about this. When I look back, it was actually an extremely stressful time in my life, and it was just a matter of survival from day to day.

A NEW PERSPECTIVE

As I mentioned earlier, this stress culminated in a major depression for me at the age of forty. I never thought this could happen to me, but it did, and I am actually grateful as I look back on this time. I knew I had to reset my priorities and accept help from my husband, children, parents, and in-laws. For a few years, my husband even put in our budget a housekeeper to come in two times a month to help out with the cleaning.

With a new and better outlook on chores, I began to see how we, as a family, could all have specific assigned chores and accomplish things together in a much quicker manner. The children were assigned duties to keep their rooms clean, keep the bathroom tidy, fold their clothes, set the table, help with dishes, and do other things to help the family.

Working with a psychiatrist, I began to feel myself again and see things in a new light. This realization changed the way I looked at many things, even the mundane things like household chores. With the entire family all chipping in and helping, I suddenly saw chores as family time and being able to accomplish things together in a shorter period of time. Once tasks were completed, it felt good to know that this was a team effort. One of the things we would do as a family, after the chores on the weekend, was reward ourselves with an outdoor family outing to one of the many beautiful parks, beaches, or trails to hike here in Hawaii.

THE FAMILY THAT WORKS TOGETHER, PLAYS TOGETHER

As the children got older, it became the tradition to do chores over the weekend together and then talk about where we would be going after. Back in the "old" days, there were not many sports groups for soccer, baseball, or flag football, so my husband and I would come up with our own family activities. When I look back, these simple activities were some of the best family times and memories I can recall. We would go bicycling, all six of us, or take after-dinner walks around the neighborhood. There would be weekend picnics at the beach, or we would just enjoy the neighborhood parks with the jungle gyms, monkey bars, and other play equipment. The kids were always the happiest when they were outdoors with us, and I know that money just would not and could not buy this.

There were times when I thought to myself, I have so many things to do at home, but I forced myself to go out with the family and have never regretted a minute of this. I always heard my elders telling me to enjoy my young children because before you know it, they will be all grown up. I could never believe this statement because when you are caring for four young children, all you can think of is "When are you going to grow up and do things for yourself?" Well, my advice is to believe it when people tell you to enjoy your children when they're young because it is true. In a blink of an eye, they are graduating high school and then perhaps college and getting married and having families of their own.

CUB SCOUTS AND BOY SCOUTS

There was a wonderful activity which entered our lives when our three boys were younger and that was Cub Scouts of America and then Boy Scouts of America. Our neighbors started this in our young neighborhood, and we finally decided to join them. This was one of the best things we ever did for our boys. We had weekly Cub Scout meetings at our home where they would learn how to cook, tie knots, and much more. We would have overnight campovers in our backyards. Even our daughter, the youngest in the family, took part in these activities we had at our home. As the boys advanced onto Boy Scouts, we continued to do the planned family activities once a month and even assisted each of the boys with their Eagle Projects. Now that my children are grown and have their own families, we have such wonderful memories of time spent together. My children never once talk about the material possessions they had but rather recall fondly the time we spent together doing things as a family. I truly believe that this ongoing connectedness keeps building day by day and helps us develop a true bond that keeps us happy and fulfilled, in good times and bad.

DANCING TOGETHER AS A FAMILY

My youngest daughter also had her own activity outlet, which was dancing. She started lessons when she was three years old under the tutelage of a sixteen-year-old teacher, Wendy Calio- Gilbert, at Sabrina Starr Dance Studios in Wahiawa. Stephen and I both had office hours on Saturday mornings, so out of necessity, we had to enroll her in something that would keep her busy on Saturdays. Fortunately, she enjoyed and thrived in dancing, and she soon brought the passion of dancing into the home.

There were times in our home, when we would just start "free dancing" to random music and not even know why we were doing it. When movement is done as a spontaneous activity, it does not really feel like exercise but rather like something to be shared with one another. I recall one incident where I heard Christmas music, and I got so excited that I started to dance, spin, and then tripped, out of control, knocking over a nearby table. We might have even had that on video, but I remember laughing so hard and having such a great time doing "free dance."

As the children grew older, they wanted to go to the gym when they were in high school, but I just could not see us spending money for that. With four healthy children, I instead asked them to consider doing extra household chores as their exercise, like car washing, yardwork, and extra cleaning. When our boys were older in high school, we had them take summer jobs at the school like helping the janitor or assisting with landscaping because this could count as exercise in real life, but this time actually accomplishing something. I heard some complaining, but I feel that overall, it made them more capable adults and helped them learn to appreciate the value of money and the little things more.

Activities in our family just seemed to naturally evolve as a way of life. We even recruited the boys to get involved in their sister's dance activities like taking part in *The Nutcracker* or helping out with making set decorations for various parades and recitals. The four children loved their sports, and soon they were all participating in volleyball or basketball. They may not have been the most outstanding players, but they sure had fun, and I thoroughly enjoyed attending their games to cheer them on. My third son enjoyed being the rebel, and instead of joining team school sports, he became a wonderful skateboarder. This love of movement and activities has continued regularly in all of their lives, even into college as well as their years as young adults. As their mother, it is so nice to see that exercise is looked on as something fun and they continue to pursue it as part of their life routines.

THE VERY BEST EXERCISE FOR EVERYONE

As I continue to get older and become more tech savvy, one of the best devices I recently purchased was a wrist pedometer. No, not the fancy Fitbit, but something I saw online for thirty dollars. This was the best investment I have ever made, and it even records my blood pressure, heart rate, and pulse. Since I am a naturally competitive person, I now track my steps daily to try to get as many steps as possible in a day. It has motivated me to challenge myself as well as others, and it reminds me to just keep walking throughout the day. When I park far away from my destination, I feel very happy to be able to get more steps in, especially if I have been sitting in front of my computer all day. If I am shopping after work, especially at large stores like Costco, I love to walk up and down the aisles just for more steps.

It has been commonly noted that 10,000 steps a day is a good estimate of steps for adults to take each day in order to achieve good health. However, in a recent study published that examined almost 17,000 women, the scientists found that the sweet spot for reducing the risk of premature death by 40 percent was 4,500 steps a day. Women who moved more definitely had less premature deaths, up to a plateau of about 7,500 steps a day. So, with my family participants, I always encourage them to count their steps and know that taking more steps is definitely better than taking fewer.

When talking about exercise, research has repeatedly shown that walking is the best exercise for all ages to partake in. There is no equipment needed, it is accessible anytime, and it has a low risk of injury. As a result, walking has the lowest dropout rate and the benefits are numerous.

Walk with a Doc – Oahu

With this information in mind, I decided to start my own local chapter of the Walk with a Doc nonprofit organization, called Walk with a Doc – Oahu. My friend and dear mentor, Dr. Annemarie Sommer, was a staunch advocate of this program and after several years of encouragement from her, I decided to bring this program to my island of Oahu. My fellow medical school classmate Dr. Craig Kadooka had already started a Walk with a Doc group in Hilo on the big island of Hawaii that met with much success, so it was time to bring it to Oahu! As you will recall, I started my free weekly community event, Walk with a Doc – Oahu, in my community, where people of all ages and fitness levels could come together and just walk with me in a nontraditional setting.

I loved this worldwide program from the moment I heard about it. The mastermind of this movement is Dr. David Sabgir, a cardiologist in Columbus, Ohio, who began this revolutionary program about fifteen years ago. He thought outside the box and asked his patients to get healthier by walking with him on a Saturday at the nearby park. This idea took off like wildfire and soon walking groups started popping up all over the United States and then to other countries. It is now in over twenty-five countries with more than five hundred walking groups all around the world.

My Walk with a Doc – Oahu group started in February 2016, and we are now moving into our fourth year of having this free weekly program at nearby Patsy T. Mink – Central Oahu Regional Park on Saturdays from 8:00 to 9:00 a.m. My walkers range in age from one to ninety-three. I know that much of the success of my weekly program is the fellowship and support we give one another each week to keep striving for good health. Just getting their shoes on and driving out at 8:00 a.m. on a Saturday morning means commitment, and I will always acknowledge that. There are so many times when I, myself, wake up on Saturday morning thinking of every excuse in the book not to go, but I do it for them. After all, I am the Doc! Once it is done, I feel so proud of myself for the effort, and it is such a great way to start off the weekend! My walkers think I am helping them, but in reality, they are the ones who are motivating me to get out there and exercise.

Hike with a Doc and Dance with a Doc

Just as an aside, since most of my walkers are fifty years and older, I heard many requests to do other activities, outside of just Walk with a Doc. In response to their requests, I initiated a new supplemental program called Hike with a Doc, which follows immediately after our Walk with a Doc program. From May to September, our seniors and other walkers enjoy exploring different nearby walking paths and routes. This proved to be a very popular and enjoyable addition, since it is always more fun to hike together in a group.

Due to the sometimes-rainy weather during our winter and spring months, I decided to stop the Hike with a Doc program during that time and replace it with Dance with a Doc, which takes place from October to April at a nearby dance studio, Pas de Deux. We recently had our very first Dance with a Doc and it was a smashing success! This free activity is also open to the public; no dance experience needed. On this last dance session, we learned the entire jazz funk dance moves to Earth, Wind & Fire's song "September" in less than an hour.

Moving More Daily – A Lifelong Goal

Incorporating movement into your life has to be a lifelong pursuit that involves creativity, purposeful intent, and fun. I have found that when activity incorporates family and friends, it is something that most of us can maintain for a lifetime. So, I now challenge you to step out and find your happy place with movement. Be daring and try a new sport or join others in different things like water aerobics, yoga, Zumba, or anything else that seems interesting to you and reap the rewards. You will be proud of yourself and your family just for trying.

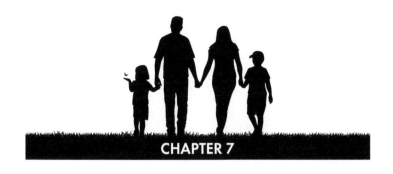

CHAPTER 7

THE INCREDIBLE VALUE OF SLEEP AND BREAKFAST

Besides nutrition and movement, there are two other very important factors that can help control our weight gain and lead to a healthier state of being. These two things are breakfast and sleep.

THE MOST IMPORTANT MEAL OF THE DAY – BREAKFAST

We have all heard it said that breakfast is the most important meal of the day. However, my experience as a pediatrician has shown me that this is definitely not the norm for the majority of the families who come in to see me.

I do believe this habit of eating breakfast is etched into our life during our young, formative years. For myself, growing up in a household of eight, my grandfather would be up at the crack of dawn tending to his vegetable garden and yard work. He would be the first to have his breakfast and then my dad would follow and make all of us a hot breakfast. It was a fun time to sit around and talk about what things would be coming up for the day. Since this was the tradition, I do not recall a single day growing up when I went without breakfast.

As a young adult in medical school and then in pediatric residency, breakfast was something I could not live without. At night, my happy time was thinking about my breakfast in the morning and look forward to it as I drifted into sleep. This habit has carried on in my life as a mother, and to this day, my adult children have continued to be great breakfast eaters.

Currently, many people skip this first meal of the day, thinking they are getting ahead on cutting calories. But the truth is that skipping breakfast actually packs on the pounds in the long run. Every morning, your body needs fuel to run on and it lets you know by making you feel extra hungry. When lunchtime hits, you are bound to eat more than if you had a satisfying breakfast or you might be tempted to raid the snack trays in your office. With breakfast, you are able to resist both these temptations.

An interesting fact is that the large, heavyweight Japanese sumo wrestlers who want to gain a very large amount of weight are not allowed to eat breakfast. This is meant to starve them and mimic starvation so that their metabolism slows down and their bodies gear up to store fat.

FAMILY MEALTIMES ARE CRUCIAL

What I want to share is that habits form at a young age. They form deep grooves in your brain and impact you later in life. Scientific studies have shown over and over the importance of eating breakfast for an energy boost, better memory, sharper focus, and, most of all, controlling appetite for the rest of the day. When you go without breakfast, it feels like you have been cheated, and by midmorning when your stomach starts to rumble, you suddenly feel the urge to grab whatever is most convenient. That quick pick-me-upper is almost never the most nutritious choice, and it is generally something sweet and starchy. This midmorning snack will satisfy you only for a short time. When lunch rolls by, you will realize that you have already had your little cheat snack, so another meal will pass. What happens to most people, especially teens, is they will be so hungry after school that they will have a very large snack or a full meal after school with their friends or at home. This, in turn, leads to feeling heavy, sluggish, and tired. They will frequently feel like taking a nap, and then when dinner swings by, it will not interest them. In the early evening hours, when hunger strikes again, they will be hitting the refrigerator for a late-night snack.

This same pattern seems to occur for many adults as well. Thus, I have seen time and time again, many college freshmen gaining that famous "Freshman fifteen," or weight gain of fifteen pounds after their first year of college.

SLEEP IS A LEARNED BEHAVIOR

So, let's back up and see how we can avoid this situation. The number-one excuse I hear from my patients for not eating breakfast is that they are too tired. My quick response to this is "Go to bed earlier." This is easier said than done. When talking about breakfast, we must talk about sleep as well because these two factors go hand in hand. Both sleep and breakfast have been shown to be two very important factors in helping people of all ages control their weight and help them perform at their maximum the next day.

In our modern world today, sleep has gotten a bad rap and has become something that we put way down on our list of priorities. As an adult, I sometimes hear my colleagues bragging about how little sleep they get, and they think that they can still perform well. But the truth is, sleep is imperative for total body restoration, muscle repair, improving your immune system, better memory storage, and just overall well-being. Study after study are now being conducted on the importance of sleep and no one can deny its importance. If you are not getting enough sleep, you are truly robbing your body of something vital for it to thrive.

Developing good and consistent sleep habits are crucial for all ages, but especially for the very young. From the first time I see newborn babies in my office, I start to talk about the importance of sleep, not only for the baby, but also for the chronically tired parents. The keys to developing great sleep habits are consistency and continued reinforcement of the rituals you do prior to sleep. What this means is whether it is a weekday or a weekend, everyone in the family strives to have a consistent ritual for bedtime, which could include brushing/ flossing teeth, reading a book, saying a prayer, talking about the day, a goodnight kiss, and then lights out. After over thirty-five years of practicing as a pediatrician, I find that for the parents who heed my advice and allow this pattern to continue, their newborn babies soon self-soothe and sleep eight to ten hours through the night by three to four months of age. The new parents I work with say it is impossible, but I have seen it over and over, and all four of my children were sleeping through the night by four months of age.

My theory is that if this works for little babies, then it can work at any age. Sleep is a learned behavior, and you can always change behavior no matter what your age. For the older children and teens whom I work with, I always tell them it is crucial that everyone understands the value of sleep and hence the urgency to get the recommended hours. By forming nighttime rituals, which everyone can be a part of, success will be more likely to occur. Again, the easiest way to do this is to set bedtimes for your kids, depending on their ages, reinforce nighttime rituals like reading or talking about the day as a family, and really trying to turn off all electronics half an hour to one hour prior to bedtime. If the adults are all in, the rest of the family will follow. The teens will know if the parents are all in by observing their behavior, so by following along, you will develop their trust. I guarantee that once the family is sleeping better, everyone will feel so much better and the likelihood of eating breakfast increases.

Sleep Recommendations

The following are the recommended hours of sleep by the National Sleep Foundation according to age, but just remember everyone's sleep needs are different:

- Ages three to five years: eleven to thirteen hours
- Ages five to twelve years: ten to eleven hours
- Adolescents: eight and a half to nine and a half hours
- Adults: seven to nine hours

Power Naps

A question I get often is the value of naps. It is important to try to not have long afternoon naps, as this may leave one too awake to fall asleep at night. Instead of very long naps of over two to three hours, during the day, if you or your child need to recharge your batteries, try a "power nap." Power naps are designed to revitalize oneself from drowsiness and should be limited to no more than twenty to thirty minutes duration. These naps should also take place before 4:00 p.m. so as not to disrupt nighttime sleep schedules.

By getting adequate sleep at night, everyone will have better ease at getting up in a better mood, feel better, and not have that foggy daytime sleepiness feeling all day. Adequate sleep will help you boost your metabolism, feel more energized to be active, and have less of a tendency to eat sweet, starchy foods throughout the day. The bottom line is getting enough sleep helps control your weight and so much more.

Be Careful about Screen Time

On another note, as we talk about sleep, I mentioned earlier that screen time is now one of the greatest robbers of sleep. It is so important to remove the temptation of all screens from your children's bedrooms. The bedroom should be associated with rest and sleep, and without the screen close by, sleep becomes much easier. Again, parents must also heed this advice and consider the same for themselves. Recent studies show that the "blue light" from our screens have an adverse effect on sleep. As a pediatrician, one of the first things I tell young parents is not to use the television or iPad as a babysitter. The American Academy of Pediatrics actually recommends zero screen time for children under three years of age. This even includes Sesame Street and the PBS television station. Studies are showing that screen time does not stimulate the young mind and, in fact, just talking, reading, and interacting with your young child will be far more beneficial in helping to develop good habits for your child later in life. Thus, my recommendation would be no television, video games, or other similar electronics in any bedrooms from the very beginning to promote sleep and overall better health habits.

HAVE A BREAKFAST BUFFET

When I was a young mother feeding my hungry family in the morning, I would frequently offer traditional breakfast foods as well as leftovers from dinner the night before. I would also lay out several different types of fruits and, yes, even vegetables, if available. There was often some lasagna, chicken, cold cereal, waffles, PBJ toast, broccoli, and much more. With the convenience of a microwave, it only takes seconds to heat up, and I learned that it was fun to think outside the box of traditional breakfast foods. I also love making all types of homemade soups that contain veggies and meats or tofu. I recall my maternal grandparents from China always had some type of soup daily for most of their meals. It was always a big surprise what was going to be laid out for that morning buffet. With a smorgasbord of food, the entire family could choose what they wanted. Whatever was left over, it would be put away for another meal or wrapped and placed in their homemade lunches.

When my kids were at school, their lunches were always a surprise, and other classmates loved to see what they had. I even recall my daughter coming home and asking me to pack a little extra fruits and veggies, as her friends wanted to try things. I think she actually made lunch an exciting event with her classmates.

IMPORTANCE OF PREPLANNING MEALS AND SNACKS

One of the keys to eating breakfast daily or preparing home lunches is preplanning. In the morning, I admit I am still in a little bit of a fog, but I have already planned in my head the night before exactly what I want to eat. With my young children, whenever I picked them up from school or after an event, I always had a cooler of fruits, veggies, and water in the car ready for them. Not only did they have a good snack, but we also saved a lot of money. Yes, we occasionally took our children to fast-food restaurants, but this was the exception.

Another great tip that I did for preplanning was using the weekend to create two or three large pots of stews, soups, or sauces for the coming week. By doing this, dinner would be ready within minutes after coming home from work. Another quick solution was using my crockpot for a great ready-to-eat hot dinner at the end of the day. When you are heating up dinner or setting the table, this is a great time to allow the children to help you make their own lunches and snacks for the next day. By doing this, everyone gets involved with the meal and snack prep, and the family members are more likely to eat what they have helped to prepare.

BABY STEP CHANGES

Sleep and breakfast have so many benefits for everyone in the family. Consider talking about this topic no matter what the age of your children. It's never too late, even for parents and grandparents, to readjust your schedule. In the next chapter, we will talk about setting small baby steps and goals as you move forward toward changing a lifetime of unhealthy habits. Remember, the slower the change is implemented, the more permanent it becomes. As I tell the families I work with all the time, if you have not cleaned your home for two or three years, don't expect to get the job completed in two or three weeks. By investing in the time and effort of making healthy changes, the rewards you reap will be multiplied for years to come.

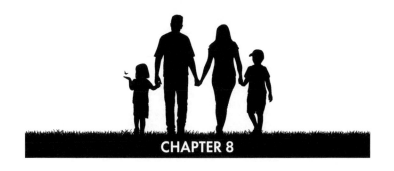

CHAPTER 8

SMALL GOALS AMOUNT TO BIG WINS

When I was a young girl, my dad had this weekly tradition of taking all four of us kids to the main public library on Friday nights to borrow books. This was the highlight of my week, as my dad worked on weeknights from Monday through Thursday. I loved to read biographies of famous people and soon found myself reading the biographies of famous women like Florence Nightingale, Madam Curie, and, finally Elizabeth Blackwell, the first woman doctor in the United States. I was so fascinated with her that at the tender age of six or seven years old, I announced to my family that I wanted to be a woman physician. This was back in the sixties, and I did not even know of a woman doctor in Hawaii, but my mind was made up that this is what I wanted to be.

As a young child, I had no clue about goal setting, but I made it a daily goal to take a step closer each day toward that goal. For example, whenever anyone needed a bandage, I would run to get it. I would always accompany my mom to visit my grandparents or sick relatives at the hospital. Whenever I saw a physician, I would picture myself already working as a physician, complete with a stethoscope around my neck and a crisp white coat on.

I wanted to start with my personal story in this chapter because it is my story on goal setting and how my crazy dream turned into reality. I will also share with you later in the chapter other techniques that have been shown to help many in setting and achieving specific goals.

GRIT MAKES THE DIFFERENCE

As a young girl who wanted to become a doctor, my family was always very encouraging, especially my dad. When other people approached me and told me this was not a good idea, it somehow gave me more fuel to prove them wrong. For many years, I can distinctly remember picturing in my mind, myself as an adult, wearing a white coat having already achieved this audacious dream of becoming a woman doctor. I lived and breathed this dream daily, in my schoolwork, my outside activities, and in everything I did. I always knew I was not the smartest person in my class, but I think I always worked the hardest. Back in my school days, the Catholic nuns gave us two grades: one for our actual work and then a second grade for effort. I know the first column was not always A's, but the second column for effort was always excellent. My dad would always ask me after a test or challenge of any sort, "Did you try your best?" I always answered with a yes, and he kept urging me to move forward.

The same approach also seemed to work with sports. At twelve years old, I learned how to play tennis and loved it. Within a year, I was on the Maryknoll High School tennis team, and I recall spending hours on the Ala Moana tennis court backboards hitting balls against a backboard for hours trying to perfect my serve or strokes. Playing a sport in high school reinforced in me the lesson of trying your best to achieve your goal and putting in the hard work daily.

YOU CAN'T FORCE ANYONE TO DO SOMETHING THEY DON'T WANT TO DO

Fast-forward to being a young, working mother with four active children and trying to apply these same rules to dealing with life's challenges. Yes, I had big goals for myself, my work, my family, and my children, but now I started realizing this is a whole new ball game. This was now not just about me, but about the other members of the family. I quickly found out that I got a lot of resistance if I forced someone to do something just because I wanted it for them. An example to illustrate this point is when my third son was in elementary school and he would bring C's home. He was a very smart young man, and I told him I knew he had a lot of potential, to which he immediately replied, "What's wrong with a C? I am an average person like most people." For me, this was a hard pill to swallow, as I was not used to my children being uncertain of their potential, not working to the best of their ability, or setting goals for the future. I always thought everyone knew from a young age what their purpose in life was and how to achieve it. This was a big reality check for me.

EVERYONE PITCHES IN

After my severe depressive episode at age forty and my husband and I finally realized that we needed the entire family to pitch in and help out with everyday chores, we divided the household chores according to age and abilities. There were daily chores as well as weekend and monthly chores. No allowance was offered for this, and it was repeated over and over in our home to our children that this is just what a family does, and this was their way of contributing to the family.

With consistency, reminders, and time, the kids slowly accepted their responsibilities and completed the tasks assigned to them. I actually think it made them feel pride in doing their little part for the family as well as learning life skills that would later prove to be very helpful as they started to live on their own.

Looking back, setting goals as a family, especially with younger children, was always a big challenge. My husband and I did not have a book or outline to follow back then, but I did want to share with you an approach that seemed to work very well for the families I worked with in our recent family workshops. This approach has been used by many over the years in all types of situations and has resulted in much success.

GOAL SETTING METHOD

This method is called the S.M.A.R.T. approach.

- **S = specific**: What exactly do you want to achieve?
- **M=measurable**: How will you know you have achieved it?
- **A= attainable**: Is it something you can control?
- **R= relevant**: Why is this applicable to your life?
- **T= time-based**: How long will it take to achieve your goals?

Families or individuals can use this method to write down a specific goal. The following is an example of a vague goal that would not work well: "I want our family to get healthier." In the family discussion, it should be more specific, like "Our family will walk together for at least fifteen minutes every day for the next two weeks." This goal is doable and definitely achievable for the entire family. And it is a way to form a good, healthy habit, and the chance of succeeding in this is greater with everyone buying in. Additionally, if the adults want to set individual goals, this could also be implemented together with the family goals. For example, if the parents want to sneak in fifteen minutes of walking after dinner, this could be piggybacked with the family goal of getting more exercise in general. If other family members are free, then they could also accompany Mom or Dad on this extra walk. It is always a good idea to write down the agreed-on family goal and place it on the refrigerator so that each family member can remind one another of getting this done daily. Psychologists now say it takes about thirty consecutive days to make a habit permanent. It makes sense to choose a new family goal at the start of every month, or at selected intervals, and review how the previous goal went.

START SMALL AND SUCCEED

Remember when you and your family are starting off on goal setting to always take small bites, not big ones. Succeeding in these smaller goals will boost your confidence for tackling the larger goals.

On a final note, taking lifestyle changes to the extreme never seems to work. I have seen some families tell me that they want to be healthier, so they immediately stop eating rice or starches completely. They do start to lose weight; however, this can only last for a limited time. Soon, they are back to old eating habits and their weights yoyo back up. It is now shown that these patterns of fluctuating weights can be more detrimental to your health, so it is vital that you make changes gradually. Keep in mind that the more gradual the change, the more permanent the change. It is going to be hard work and there are going to be days when you don't feel like it, but keep pressing on and invest in your future success. Keep your eye on the goal and the rewards that will come.

When I was a young girl, my dad taught me a portion of a poem by Henry Wadsworth Longfellow. I recited it and thought of it so many times that I committed it to my memory. I even used it as my comment under my senior photo, and it goes like this:

> *"The heights great men have achieved and kept,*
> *Were not attained by a single flight,*
> *But they while their companions slept,*
> *Were toiling upward through the night"*

This poem was instrumental in encouraging me to push forward on what seemed at times like an impossible dream: to become a woman physician back in the seventies. Despite failures and disappointments along the way, I knew that it would take hard work and perseverance to accomplish this goal. I feel blessed to have had the help from many mentors, and I now try to pay it forward by being that mentor to high school, premed, medical students, and residents as they move along their own personal journeys.

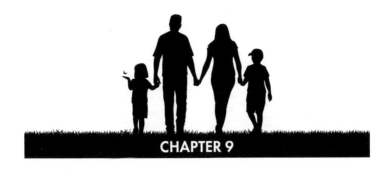

CHAPTER 9

LIFE IS ABOUT BEING IN THE PRESENT MOMENTS

It is sometimes fun to look back and recall carefree childhood memories. One of the first things that came to my mind was how happy and free I felt as a young girl when I went roller-skating for hours up and down the street I lived on. I can recall the cracks in the sidewalks, the houses I passed by, and the details of my neighbors' houses and yards. Without knowing it, I was savoring every moment of joy that filled me and it was and will always be my very happy place from childhood.

As a young, busy mother, there were so many things to do that I felt like I missed being present in many moments with my kids. I was always thinking of the future tasks and worrying about whether I made the right decisions in the past. I recall looking at my youngest one day when she was four years old and wondering to myself, "How did you grow up so quickly?" It is sometimes even harder for me to remember the details of my children when they were growing up. I am just happy to know that they are decent human beings despite all the mishaps and mistakes my husband and I may have made. The few moments that I do remember are the times when I could really focus on them and enjoy that special time being fully present with each one of them.

Social media robs our time. In today's quick-paced world, one cannot help but be caught up in all this busyness. Our social media on our smart phones, tablets, computers, and other electronics keep showing us what others are doing, the many activities available to us, and much more at the touch of a button. Sometimes, we spend so much time scrolling through social media that by the time we decide to do something, one hour has passed.

Practice being present 100 percent of the time. In our recent workshops with parents, I learned some practical tips for living in this so-called present moment. It has opened my eyes to a better way of living my life with more joy and fulfillment. By focusing on the present activity I am doing, I am not thinking of the past or the future. At times, I will not even take out my phone camera to take vacation photos but instead just savor where I am, who I am with, and what I am feeling, taking in all that I can at that moment. This has given me a better recall of the memory. Of course, this is something new for me, and I am trying to practice it daily.

Nowadays when I am at work and seeing patients, I take a deep breath when touching the doorknob to open the door and try to clear my mind so that I can be fully present to the patient in front of me. Recently, it has also helped me slow down my eating. Due to having a busy schedule my entire life, I realized that I became conditioned to shovel food down my throat in the shortest time possible. It seemed to be something I was proud of, but as I examined this habit, I realized it was leading to me overeat many times and not appreciate the full eating experience. By taking the time to deliberately slow down my eating and even taking at least eight to ten bites per mouthful, while putting my fork down, I am able to feel the texture of the food; appreciate the smell, appearance, and taste; and be fully aware of this meal. I also found that by eating this way, I could be aware of feeling full and understanding when I should stop.

HELP EACH OTHER BE MINDFUL

Another advantage to being fully present for many of our workshop participants was the fact that you become very aware of your impulses and what your weak points are. A personal example of this is my awareness of my love of ice cream. If I know I have ice cream in my freezer, then it becomes very difficult to resist it as a snack at night. A solution I came up with was to simply not buy a half gallon carton in my home freezer and instead eat a fruit or just brush my teeth, call it a day and go to bed. By understanding this, you can then manage your own environment so that this impulse will not be acted on or avoided totally.

For young children, their brains are not fully developed, so they will need the help of their parents, grandparents, or other adults to remind them to be mindful, which can lead to better decision-making.

One of the techniques that my husband and I used with our kids for discipline was the well-known "timeout." Timeouts were used for specific reasons, such as if our child did something to hurt themselves or others, this was a definite timeout. The length of the timeouts was determined by our child's age. For example, if our child was ten years old, they would have to sit in the boring timeout corner for ten minutes. The rule of thumb was one minute for each year of life. Overall, we found this to be quite effective, and when looking back on this, I now see that this gave our children quiet time to reflect on what brought them there in the first place.

MEDITATION: THE PAUSE BUTTON

When my husband and I were raising our four children back in the eighties and nineties, we always had "quiet time" on Sunday afternoon, when everyone would simply lie down for an hour to rest and take a break. We also utilized a technique called "time-outs" whenever the children did acts that could have hurt themselves or others. The whole point of these time-outs was to have the child sit in a quiet corner and reflect on what misdeed they had just committed.

The current terminology or trendy word that we now use is *meditation*. From doing our recent family workshops, I can see the many benefits meditation has in helping people of all ages. Taking even a few moments to get in touch with where you are or how you are feeling can help you make better decisions moving forward. At work, if things start getting hectic and I am falling behind in the schedule, I simply take a few seconds to breathe, regroup, and remind myself to be 100 percent present on every new patient I am seeing that day. This has helped me tremendously in listening fully to the patient or parents and in making the right decisions and choices. As with any new habit, this skill does take time and practice to develop.

Practice Belly Breathing

One of the homework assignments that was very helpful for our families was choosing and practicing one of the many free meditation resources available online. One of their favorites was "belly breathing" to help calm, destress, and relax, instantly. This is performed by placing a stuffed animal on your tummy and then lying down comfortably for a few minutes and watching your belly go up and down as you concentrate on this and nothing else. I have been doing this recently, especially when I have so many thoughts rushing through my head at night. I start belly breathing three to four times and really focusing on my breathing. By doing this often, I generally find myself immediately falling asleep. The beauty of this is that almost anyone of any age can be successful at this.

Meditation can help you calm down and reconnect with your desire to be healthier. It can also help you focus and make better decisions in a more disciplined manner. I am still new to all of this, but I see the success in others and will continue to practice this.

Once again, every person and family is different and unique. If belly breathing doesn't work for you, try a different meditation technique. Practicing mindfulness and meditation can be something the entire family can practice together, and I believe it could lead to a more harmonious life.

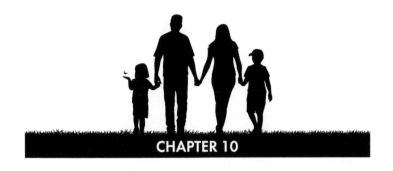

CHAPTER 10

A POSITIVE ATTITUDE CHANGES EVERYTHING

BE KIND TO YOURSELF AND OTHERS

The process of changing one's lifetime habits is not easy. We always start out striving to do the best that we can to accomplish the goals we set, but the truth is, we are bound to make mistakes. Here is a big secret: you are human, and none of us are perfect. My hope is that you don't condemn yourself or others for these moments of weakness or mishaps.

For some reason, your brain always wants to pay attention and focus on the negatives rather than the positives. It is so much easier to come down on negative behavior in ourselves or others, and it's difficult to point out the positives when they occur. In my mind and experience, I know this, but to actually pick each other up and point out times when you or others are doing something positive is rare.

GIVE PRAISE FREELY

As a pediatrician, this is advice that I give young parents all the time. I remind them to pay close attention to the positive behaviors their child is doing and reward this instead of their negative behavior. For example, if your child is reacting positively to the new baby who was brought home, say something about this. If you don't, your child will try to get your immediate reaction by doing something they were told not to do.

Practicing this attitude of gratitude, you will be able to make this positive behavior more likely to occur in the future. Examples of praise or positive feedback could include: "I saw that you chose the apple instead of the Oreo cookies…good choice" or "You're right. I did not walk the dog tonight. Would you like to join me?". When we give someone positive feedback for a specific behavior, that person is more likely to do that behavior again because of the positive feeling that came with it.

The receiver of positive praise not only benefits, but the giver of the positive comment benefits as well. Studies show that those who give positive praise are happier in the moment, but studies have shown that this happiness continues for the giver for months to follow. By getting into the habit of writing thank you notes or a sentence or two in a gratitude journal, you will become so much more aware of the good and abundance in your life. More research is coming out that practicing gratitude changes your entire outlook on life and improves your sleep, disposition, and immune system.

THE VALUE OF RELATIONSHIPS

When we talk about being grateful, it is always a good idea to teach our children to focus on the relationships they have in their lives rather than the material things or occurrences. In this day and age of high credit card debt for many millennials, we need to prioritize what is most important in our lives, and ultimately, these are the close relationships we form over the years.

As our young children were growing up, my husband and I struggled financially while growing our private practices. We decided that we would not buy brand name shoes or clothes for ourselves and the children, and we held out for as long as possible when it came to subscribing to cable TV. We always got pushback from our two older boys, but they learned to live with this. Today, when my adult children and I look back on those good old days, we only talk about the great memories we shared doing things as a family, and the topic of generic brand clothes or other things rarely comes up.

MOVE INTO A PROBLEM-SOLVING MODE

Another additional benefit of having a constant attitude of gratitude is that it removes you from being in a complaining or whining mode and keeps you constantly prepared in a solution-seeking mode. For example, when the new water park first opened up, our children all wanted to go, but this was way over our budget at the time. As a result, we sat down as a family and told them to offer up other ideas or activities we could do together. Since we are so lucky to live in Hawaii, the natural solution was to simply have a beach day, which was completely free and just as much fun. As a family, you are more likely to come up with a mutually agreed-on solution. Everyone feels happier for this process and it develops skills for our children to utilize in the future as adults.

BE KIND TO EVERYONE

In this home atmosphere of gratitude, the environment should be more conducive to speaking kindlier to one another and expressing gratefulness. Sometimes, the people we love the most are the ones whom we are not so nice to because there is a comfort zone there. They are family and will love you no matter how you speak or treat them; however, when you are trying to cultivate those warm, fuzzy, close relationships, it never hurts to try extra hard to be cordial and courteous, just like you would behave with a stranger. The more you practice in the home, the more likely you will take this attitude to your workplace or school. This attitude of gratitude can be quite contagious, so share it everywhere you go, even with strangers.

COUNT YOUR BLESSINGS

In many ways, having this type of positive attitude of abundance is about being mindful of the many blessings you have in this wonderful country of ours. We take living in the United States for granted. I recall conversations I had with my maternal grandparents from China, who immigrated to this foreign land called Hawaii. They came across the Pacific Ocean seeking a better life and had heard of the many great opportunities here. They were laborers and had no formal education, but within one generation, my mother went to colleges on the mainland and received her master's degree in social work in the 1940s. I am so grateful to my grandparents from China and appreciate their courage and sacrifice to seek a better life in a new foreign land. Even though our country is currently going through some turbulent times, I still believe it is the greatest country in the world, and I am so grateful to be a United States citizen.

One of the best ways to appreciate all the blessings you have is to write them down in a daily gratitude journal. Acknowledging one or two things that you are grateful for daily can help prepare and strengthen you to deal with tough situations when they arise. It is a simple way to focus your attention on the positive things in your life. By writing in a gratitude journal, you are forcing yourself to tune in to the good things in your life, which you might otherwise take for granted. Scientific studies in positive psychology now prove that a gratitude journal not only helps you record your memories and find self-expression but is also good for your health. The conclusions of the studies show that journaling helps reduce stress, improve immune function, keep your memory sharp, boost your mood, and strengthen emotional function. As a family activity, consider doing a daily gratitude journal and share your daily excerpts with one another. You can also use your daily excerpts during "family talk about the day" time and have each family member share the one thing they are grateful for that day.

Engaging the entire family into frequent discussions of gratefulness will not only make everyone happier but also draw everyone closer to see all the good things happening in everyone's lives. When you see the abundance, you cannot help but feel contented with what you already have. At the end of our lives, we are not going to wish we had more things, but rather we will be grateful for the strong relationships we have cultivated over the years with our family and friends.

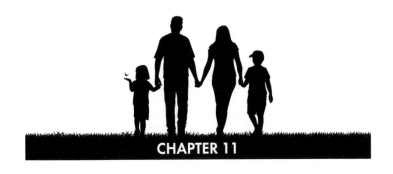

CHAPTER 11

KEEP THE PASSION BURNING

HAVE A WINNING MINDSET

From the time I was very young, I was always very competitive. I always liked to win, perhaps because I was the second child yearning for the attention of my parents or because I was sandwiched between two brothers. Whether it was in school or outdoors on the playground, I tried my best to win, and generally, I did succeed. The problem with this is once people know what you are capable of, they expect to see the same result over and over. So, in my younger years, I felt like an average person who just tried harder than most, always hoping people would not find out. This proved to be a pretty good philosophy, and my dad definitely helped reinforce it throughout my life.

MY ROLE MODEL

My dad was such an inspiration in my life. His parents, my paternal grandparents, immigrated to the United States from China and settled in Hawaii in the early 1900s. With very little English and education, they both somehow managed to start a small store business in the Palama district of Honolulu. My dad told me stories of how my grandparents would wake up early in the morning to bake little pork buns called *manaupua* and then carry large containers of these on their shoulders around the parks and neighborhood, yelling out, "Manaupua for sale!" This hard work paid off and helped them raise my dad, as well as his four brothers and one older sister.

My dad was very fortunate to attend a young men's Catholic school, St. Louis High School, and he gained a wonderful education at this men's only Catholic institution. Dad never officially had his graduation ceremony because World War II was in full swing, and on June 14th, one day after he turned eighteen years old, he signed up for the U.S. Army. He was assigned to desk duties and never saw any of the action on the combat field, as the war ended soon after he enlisted. With the G.I. Bill after his service, my dad was accepted to an East Coast college, the Massachusetts Institute of Technology. Many of his classmates also attended other Ivy League colleges, like Harvard, but my dad felt happy to be at MIT. He received his master's in civil engineering, specializing in structural engineering, a new field of expertise just starting out at the time.

I remember my dad telling stories of how he was not the smartest student, but he really tried his best. He was my role model, and I admired the courage, persistence, and dedication he had. As a young girl, I knew anything was possible if you tried. I was always of the mind-set that no matter what the outcome, if I did my best, I would have no regrets.

This shaped the way I approached everything in my life. I truly believe that to have and maintain success, talent is only a small part of the equation. Instead, hard work, perseverance, and determination is 90 percent of the answer.

PARENTS ARE THE KEY TO SUCCESS

At the family workshops I have conducted over the years, I am always so proud of my participants who have diligently attended sessions, did their homework, and achieved many of the goals they set out for themselves and their families. I then feel the hardest part is at hand: maintaining sustained success. Whenever I see my patients and their families in the office or out and about, I always love to ask how things are going. This answer ultimately depends on how engaged and involved the parents are. The children are still young and do not fully grasp the lifetime benefits of their new healthy habits. So, as parents or guardians of the family, it is imperative that the adults continue to take the lead.

This is where the family talk times that you have established must be continued on a weekly or, preferably, daily basis. Communication is key in reminding one another of the family goal of the week or month as well as in hearing the progress other members are making along the way. Accountability, even by the children, is a good motivator to keep the adults on their toes.

I remember our "talk about the day" family discussions every night where everyone in the family member could feel free to bring up any topic for discussions. I never knew what topics would be brought up. Some examples are when my children brought up why they were the only ones in the neighborhood not getting allowances, the unfairness of assigned chores, permission to extend the bedtime hours, and on and on.

I sometimes dreaded these "talk about the day" sessions because they could last a long time, depending on the topic. I would be so tired and have a million things to do, but as I look back on these family discussions, it was really one of the few times of the day when we could really get back in touch as a family and feel the connectedness. As the parents and leaders of the family, we would always end our discussions with "We will take this under advisement," but nothing was promised. My husband and I would later sit down and talk about the recent discussion and if it made sense to make adjustments where needed, especially when the children became older. The point is that when these family discussions are a regular part of the daily routine, everyone will feel that their input is valuable and trust and respect will be gained. With four children, it was always a challenge to allow the older kids more privileges, but they had to earn them and prove themselves worthy of them.

Over the years, being a parent has been an on-the-job learning experience that neither medical school nor pediatric residency prepared me for. But this I know for sure: regular communication and family talk time keeps everyone in touch and much happier. Therefore, as time marches on, stop, pause, and reflect on the steady progress everyone is making on this journey of change to healthier habits. If someone is standing out and leading the charge with exceptional progress, recognize it and reward it. It is so easy to get down on oneself or others when they fail or mess up, but be mindful of the positive behaviors and progress. Again, this takes time to focus on the present moment, especially when you are in one of these family talks. It is so easy to start drifting to the future things to do or looking back on the past regrets, but once you are listening and contributing as the leader, the children will know and appreciate your undivided attention.

BUILDING MEMORIES FOR A LIFETIME

It is funny how memories work. As I look back on those times as a young, overwhelmed, working mom, I quickly recall the feelings of the happy times we all had as a family. Things like family bike riding, family trips, staycations, Easter egg hunts, Christmases spent, and many more family activities. I know that there were many days of fatigue, worry, trying to balance the tight budget, tense discussions on how we should spend our money, and much more, but the bottom line is what really mattered was the relationships, bonding, and memories we had as a family unit. This was the glue that helped us get through tough times. Once again, it was the perseverance, hard work, and routines we established that helped each one of us succeed. I know that it can work for you and your family, too.

There were so many times when my husband and I questioned if we were parenting correctly. The children were all so different, and we always had to be flexible and adapt yet still be consistent. We simply wanted them to grow up to be hard-working, kind, and respectful individuals who would be able to contribute to society and make it a better place as adults. I am happy to report that I think we did, for the most part, accomplish this task, and now that they are all in their thirties, it feels good to say mission accomplished. I try to share with the friends and families I work with that children are truly a gift from God, but they are only on loan to us for a short time. During the time they are with us, it is our responsibility to shape them into well-controlled and disciplined adults. It is only then that they will become the best they can be and ultimately be happy and fulfilled individuals.

But just like everything worthwhile in life, it takes the daily determination and patience to see the results you strive for. My parting thought is to continue to work hard as a family and never quit. Your family is depending on you to lead the way. When you have times of messing up, know that there is always another day to start all over. I can tell you from experience that your children will thank you later for setting the boundaries, spending the time talk to them, and most of all, not giving up on them or yourself.

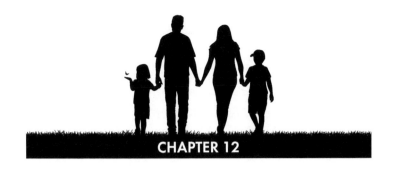

CHAPTER 12

OOPS, WE ARE ONLY HUMAN

OBSTACLES ARE WITH YOU AT EVERY SEASON IN YOUR LIFE

As a young, optimistic, premedical student at the University of Hawaii at Manoa, I was suddenly thrust into a huge culture shock. As a freshman, I sat in large, theater-style rooms, sometimes filled with 100 to 200 students. Since I graduated from Maryknoll High School, a small, private, Catholic high school with classes of no more than twenty-five students, this was a totally new experience for me. Everywhere I turned, it seemed like everyone wanted to be a doctor.

The first semester in college was brutally difficult, and there were several times when I confided in my dad that I wanted to quit. Through encouragement from family and friends who believed in me, I somehow managed to adjust and survive despite the many obstacles. At the age of twenty, I was blessed to be accepted to the UH John A. Burns

School of Medicine with "early decision" at the start of my third year as a college senior. I felt so relieved to be on my way and fulfilling my life goal. But life has a funny way of presenting you with new and even bigger obstacles.

That first year of medical school was another year of major adjustments. We were in classes from 8:00 a.m. to 5:00 p.m., and massive amounts of information were fed to us daily. We also spent many hours in the anatomy lab, dissecting our cadavers and studying late into the evenings. We even put on a white coat in our first year of medical school and had to act like real doctors and see patients. These were just a few of the many things expected of us in that first grueling year. It seemed like there was an exam every week, and I tried to keep up with everyone else. My classmates were wonderful, and we all helped one another, but I swear I had never met so many incredibly intelligent people all gathered together in this one class.

After this first traumatic semester, I went to the dean of students, Dr. Benjamin Young, to tell him that maybe medicine was really not for me. Thankfully, he told me that many students feel this way and urged me to push through. Each year that followed in medical school presented new challenges, but I kept my ultimate lifetime goal in mind and kept plodding forward. As my career moved forward, bigger and bigger obstacles kept presenting themselves continually, even after medical school. Just when you thought you got through the worst of it, you realize that you have not seen anything yet.

And so, it was, at the start of my pediatric residency training at Columbus Children's Hospital that I was now officially a physician, but there was so much to learn and experience. I was on call every third night, witnessed death every week, assumed many responsibilities that required split-second decisions, and much more. There is no question that I learned a lot, but even more surprises were lining up for me as I opened up my private practice office in Gentry Waipio, Oahu, with my husband and business partner.

I share this story with you to tell you that anything worth fighting for will not be easy. I have learned over time that you have to invest time, effort, and hard work daily. I found that keeping your goal clearly in your mind helps you to take each day one by one. In other words, don't quit, show up daily, and seek help and encouragement from others around you. Many years ago, a politician made the saying popular that "it takes a village" to help raise a child. I now look back and see how many family and friends helped me on my personal journey even when I felt like quitting. To these people who truly believed in me, I will be forever grateful.

STAY FOCUSED

Never forget that obstacles will seek you at every opportunity, so keep your goals clearly pictured in your mind. Stay focused on your daily tasks and look at problems that come up as opportunities to learn and problem solve. When you have that winning mind-set, you become that winner. Little victories each week will boost your confidence that you are one step closer to your ultimate goal of better health. Keep everyone engaged with the food planning, shopping, and prepping, so that you will not succumb to the easier and more convenient microwave of fast foods. As parents, keep the excitement going by including fresh, new ideas. Every week, sit down and choose a new recipe and get everyone involved in the shopping, prepping, and cooking. Start a new garden and try planting herbs or another vegetable like lettuce. Have a friendly competition within your family to see who can walk the most steps over the weekends. Remember, don't read every single health article or fad diet that comes up in the magazines or social media, but just stay with the basic information you have learned in this program. Remember, moderation is a good word to have and say it often, as it allows you to reward yourself every now and then.

PICK EACH OTHER UP

Everyone should be reminded of conducting the daily family talks and discussing the ongoing progress each person is making. If someone starts losing interest, reel them back in. This might be the perfect time for everyone to go over the goal setting chapter or simply sit down and have a family session where everyone can share where they are at. Perhaps a new goal could be set or a new family activity could be reintroduced to keep the momentum pushing forward. Again, the magic of this program is that no one is alone in this journey, and if someone is struggling, pick them up and be a source of encouragement. When I conducted these family sessions in my office, I tried to remind everyone at each session that they should expect days when they just don't feel like doing anything healthy. Remember, it is not about feeling like doing it, it is about the actions we take.

THE FIVE SECOND RULE

I recently came across a novel way of getting over the hurdle of doing something, even when you do not "feel" like it. I have actually tried it myself many times, and it has made me accomplish goals I never thought were possible. This is called the "Five Second Rule" by Mel Robbins and has proven to be very successful for many people over the years. No, this is not the rule where if a piece of food falls down on the floor and is picked up in less than five seconds, you may still eat it. Instead, this rule keeps us from hesitating and instead catapults us into action. Our brains are wired to avoid doing things that seem scary, difficult, or frightening, so the moment you hesitate, your brain wakes up to magnify the problem. This is known as the spotlight effect, and it takes less than five seconds to occur. Therefore, by counting backward – five, four, three, two, one – your brain has no time to stop you, and you immediately catapult into action.

By using this five-second rule, you can now go from idea to action. You know clearly what you want, the goal is in mind, and the only thing left to do is to push forward with courage and positivity. By using this five-second rule, you force yourself to be in the present moment, not regretting the past and not worrying about the future. It empowers you to feel excited about taking the right action and putting the real enemy, fear, aside. The "Five Second Rule" by Mel Robbins is one of the top ten Ted Talks ever viewed, and this method of moving into action is used worldwide. In one of my workshops, one of my families utilized this technique to do a daily family walk. There was never a day when every single family member felt like walking, but they all shouted out "5, 4, 3, 2, 1" in unison and everyone put on their shoes and went walking. When this walk was completed, they all felt so proud of themselves for accomplishing what seemed like an almost impossible task.

Remember, you are in control of the thoughts and actions in your life. You just have to decide what are the most important things to do today and get it done. Using the five-second rule helps you to stay hyper aware and focused on your present goal. If you want to make changes now, you must beat the fear that is real and in front of you. Instead of thinking fear, think of excitement and challenge. As adults, we are responsible for "parenting ourselves" because no one is going to tell us what we need to do. Once we understand this and accept the challenge, we can move forward toward making our dreams come true.

THE SECRET OF A LIFETIME OF SUCCESS

This journey you are taking toward better health is not an easy one and will require hard work. In a recent study put out by Angela Lee Duckworth, she talks about her search to find the key components of being successful. She wanted to find the secret to success and looked at graduates of West Point, Ivy League schools, spelling bee winners, successful businessmen, and many others from a wide range of fields. Her conclusion was grit and self-control were the two most important predictive variables in their real-world performances. Thomas Edison is quoted as saying that "genius is mostly just perspiration." The conclusion is that our most important talent in life is working hard, not giving up, and practicing even when it does not feel like fun. Another way of looking at this is you need to develop mental toughness in achieving any goals in your life. Thus, mental toughness is built daily through your small wins, like a muscle being challenged and growing every day. We need to remember to focus on small habits, be consistent, stick to the schedule and forget about the results. When you slip up, pick yourself up and get back on track. If you can be consistent in this thinking, you can accomplish anything.

SEEKING THE HELP YOU NEED

One final note to close this chapter on obstacles and roadblocks. As someone who has personally been through two major depressive episodes in my life, I never thought in a million years that this would happen to me. This is a real illness, and just like any other illness, there is no shame in getting the help you need. This is my plea to you: if you are feeling extreme sadness and loss of interest in life, please do not take this lightly. This could be more than just the "blues." It could be depression, especially if it is causing you problems in your day-to-day activities. Depression is not a weakness and you cannot simply snap out of it. Pick up your phone now to make an appointment to see your doctor or a mental health professional.

If you think you might hurt yourself or attempt suicide, call 9-1-1 or your local emergency number. The National Suicide Prevention Lifeline number in the United States is 1-800-273-8255 (1-800-273-TALK).

Remember, your life matters and there is help and hope for you. Reach out and call a loved one, friend, or the National Suicide Prevention Lifeline for help.

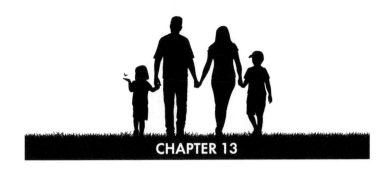

CHAPTER 13

EXCEPTIONAL FAMILY HEALTH FOR LIFE

WORKING PARENTS CAN SUCCEED

After conducting many group sessions and speaking individually in my office with my patients and their families over the years, I have found that the most rewarding part for me was to witness not only physical health improvements for everyone in the family, but also the family unit becoming stronger and thriving once again. As a practicing pediatrician for over thirty-five years, I have seen firsthand the gradual breakdown of the most essential unit in our society: the family unit. Working parents are trying their very best to keep it all together, however I feel that our environment and technology have greatly influenced our lifestyles. My hope is that you come back together as a family with this program and feel the connectedness when you work as a team. Together, everyone will be able to achieve not only health goals but also better emotional well-being.

During many sessions with parents, I have been privileged to witness improved communication and appreciation for each other. Not only does this make all family members happy, but the children now also see their parents working together as united leaders of their family. There is no longer any confusion of expectations or schedules, as everything is clear and now daily schedules are done out of habit. Mealtimes and bedtimes become enjoyable family talk times, and everyone looks forward to coming home in the evening and spending time with one another.

The leaders of the family, the parents or guardians, now feel excited about their responsibilities and the results they are seeing with just these small changes. When the children see your excitement, they become excited as well. I like to call this excitement or enthusiasm "passion."

John Maxwell, who has written many books on leadership, once said, "A great leader's courage to fulfill his vision comes from passion, not position." I want each and every one of you leaders to get up each day thinking of new and different ways to achieve goals of getting yourself and your family healthier. Your family is unique, so set goals that make sense for you and your family. When you move into action, show your family your energy, positivity, and passion. It will be very contagious and soon everyone will want to follow you.

DREAM BIG ONE STEP AT A TIME

I know that attempting a program like this is extremely intimidating and the results may be uncertain. Instead, I want you to do whatever you can to dream big, begin now, and be bold. Courage is doing what you are afraid of doing. With the knowledge that each new day is a new beginning, you can take that first step boldly and confidently. I know what it feels like – I have been there, paralyzed in that fear mode. With the help of many, I am truly living the life I was meant to live.

There is a well-known Chinese saying, "A journey of a thousand miles begins with the first step." This is so true for any journey we take. By taking small steps for continual improvement every day, eventually they will all add up and become bigger things. However, you must be patient and give it time. The secret is to take small, itty, bitty steps that will eventually lead to those giant leaps. When you take small baby steps, you cannot fail, and your mind will want to keep trying a new goal. By engaging in the small goals, your brain will bypass the fear and then become engaged because it seeks success once again. So, let's all become optimistic in our belief that we all have the potential for continual improvement if we do it slowly and consistently.

OPPORTUNITIES TO LEARN AND GROW

As you start to connect more and more as a family, you will learn to welcome and embrace challenges as new opportunities for everyone to learn something new. When things are not going the way you want them to, don't stay helpless; take action. Taking action turns worry into positive, focused energy. Be flexible and expect results to go your way. Your success in life will depend on how you deal with your failures. So, continue to be passionate about your goals and constantly strive to reach higher each time.

PAY IT FORWARD

Finally, I encourage all of the families I work with to share their newfound knowledge, success, and secrets for improved health with others they meet. In other words, pay it forward. Now that you have been given insight into better health as a family, give it away freely. Clearly, we influence one another, and you will now become a powerful motivator for others you come in contact with. You are now the one who encourages others by doing better yourself each day. The more you help others, the more I believe you will continue to help yourself and your family. This becomes a win-win for everyone, and it all starts with you.

THE NEW FAMILY REVOLUTION

I believe we are in a new revolution to return to the family unit. By strengthening this unit once again, you will not only enjoy better health but also better emotional and spiritual well-being. The problem is only a few of us are aware of this and many families don't get it yet. My hope and dream are that you and your family stay together and keep spreading the word until we flip this unhealthy trend. Let us cherish our families and show everyone what a powerful and positive source they can be, especially in shaping our children. The family revolution has started with you, and I hope we can soon burst out and change the world for the better, one family at a time. Won't you join me in this happy, healthy revolution?

ACKNOWLEDGMENTS

I would like to acknowledge several important individuals and groups who have helped me along this journey toward the completion of my book.

First, I would like to thank my dear husband, Martin M. Arinaga, for his love and support in all my new adventures these past seven years. You are a constant source of encouragement and always see the potential in me, even when I do not. Most of all, you have deepened my relationship with God, and I am so blessed to have you at my side in life.

Thank you to my pastor, Jerry Higashi, for being my spiritual support. I appreciate your prayers and words of encouragement, especially during my times of despair. Your unexpected hospital visits and talks have helped me immensely.

Thank you to my dear monthly grief support group, especially Pastor J. P., Sandra, Charlie, and Donna, for being there and helping me through my grief journey these past nine years.

To my hardworking office staff, Danielle, Kristen, and Lori, thank you for all the late nights and extra time you have given to help me. I could not have done it without your daily encouragement and deep belief in my movement.

To AlohaCare Health Insurance and the AlohaCare Community Intervention Program WaiWai Ola Grant, I thank you for honoring me as one of your 2019 grantees. Without your support of the Hawaii Healthy Family Revolution Sessions, none of this would have been possible. Thank you for investing and believing in me. A special thank-you to Sara and Stella for helping me throughout this entire process. Together, we will continue to accomplish much and greatly improve the health of Hawaii, one family at a time.

To Dr. Derrin Fukuda, psychologist, and Justin Shigematsu, certified personal trainer, thank you for all your input into the sessions and your enthusiastic participation at all the sessions.

Thank you to UHA Health Insurance, its fantastic marketing department, and an especially big thank-you to the CEO, Howard Lee, for having the foresight to see the possibilities of new innovative programs. I appreciate your generous support of my nonprofit organization, Walk with a Doc – Oahu, as well as Hike with a Doc and now Dance with a Doc these past four years. Together, we will continue to make a profound, positive impact in many lives.

To Queens Akoakoa Physician Organization, for the privilege and honor of being your Pediatric Program direc tor as well as for your support in my community outreach projects. You have been vital in helping me get the word out to our physicians as well as to our communities. Special thanks to Whitney, Ashley, Emily, Valerie, and Lara, as well as to Susan Murray, CEO of Queens Medical Center West, for all your support.

To Walk with a Doc National Headquarters in Columbus, Ohio, especially to CEO Dr. David Sabgir and his hardworking staff, Rachel, Bryan, and Gina, as well as my dear mentor, friend, and avid Walk with a Doc supporter Dr. Annemarie Sommer, thank you for showing me what a few committed individuals can do to change the world. I love being a part of your Walk with a Doc team and movement to better the health of the world.

Thank you to my grandparents, parents, and siblings, who have loved me unconditionally and have sacrificed so much for me, I appreciate and am grateful for all of it.

To my four beautiful children – David and his wife, Cheree; Chris and his wife, Samantha; Bradley; and (Stephanie) Malia – thank you for your love and support, especially after the sudden and unexpected death of Dad. I am truly grateful for being blessed with the four of you, even though you drove me crazy at times. I know that Dad would have been so proud of the caring, young adults you have become. I know I am. Special thanks to my eldest son, David, for immediately stepping up and helping me get my private practice back up and thriving again these past nine years.

Last, but not least, I give thanks to my awesome God for his bountiful blessings. Even in my darkest days, you have been there with me, and I will continue to give you thanks and praise always. Your love endures forever, and your faithfulness continues through all generations. Let me continue to be your instrument of hope and love for others.

THANK YOU

_____

Thank you so much for completing my book, *The Happy, Healthy Revolution*. I am so proud of you and hope your journey towards better health and thriving as a family continues for a lifetime.

To keep the passion alive for your entire family, continue to revisit areas in this book that seem especially challenging. This journey that you are all embarking on will not happen overnight, so be patient, encourage one another, and above all, don't give up!

My hope and dream are that your entire family will not only enjoy improved health, but also better emotional and spiritual well-being. This modern revolution of returning back to the family unit has begun with you; now get out and share it with others! Together we can change the world, one family at a time.

ABOUT THE AUTHOR

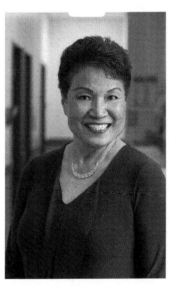

DR. THERESA Y. WEE is a pediatric health and wellness expert who has been in private practice at the Wee Wellness Center for thirty-five years. She is a graduate of the University of Hawaii John A. Burns School of Medicine and went on to complete her pediatric internship, residency, and ambulatory fellowship at Columbus Children's Hospital at Ohio State University.

Dr. Wee was born and raised in Hawaii and has a strong commitment to improving the health of the people there. Her non-profit organization, Walk with a Doc – Oahu, recently celebrated its third anniversary. She meets weekly at nearby Central Oahu Regional Park to educate, exercise, and encourage people to take that their first step towards better health. She recently helped to start the monthly Walk with a Future Doc at the University of Hawaii Medical School as well as Dance with a Doc. She has also been conducting Family Obesity Sessions over the years to help families prevent and address childhood obesity.

She is a Board Member of the Hawaii 5210, Let's Go program and a member of the American Academy of Pediatrics Hawaii chapter Childhood Obesity Committee. She also serves as the pediatric program director for the Queen's Akoakoa Physician Organization and has been providing monthly television health tips on the Take 2 Program as well as numerous other radio broadcasts.

In her spare time, she enjoys traveling and spending time with her four grown children and four grandchildren. Her hobbies include water aerobics, swimming, hiking, and cooking.

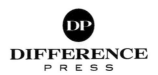

ABOUT DIFFERENCE PRESS

Difference Press is the exclusive publishing arm of The Author Incubator, an educational company for entrepreneurs – including life coaches, healers, consultants, and community leaders – looking for a comprehensive solution to get their books written, published, and promoted. Its founder, Dr. Angela Lauria, has been bringing to life the literary ventures of hundreds of authors-in-transformation since 1994.

A boutique-style self-publishing service for clients of The Author Incubator, Difference Press boasts a fair and easy-to-understand profit structure, low-priced author copies, and author-friendly contract terms. Most importantly, all of our #incubatedauthors maintain ownership of their copyright at all times.

LET'S START A MOVEMENT WITH YOUR MESSAGE

In a market where hundreds of thousands of books are published every year and are never heard from again, The

Author Incubator is different. Not only do all Difference Press books reach Amazon bestseller status, but all of our authors are actively changing lives and making a difference.

Since launching in 2013, we've served over 500 authors who came to us with an idea for a book and were able to write it and get it self-published in less than 6 months. In addition, more than 100 of those books were picked up by traditional publishers and are now available in book stores. We do this by selecting the highest quality and highest potential applicants for our future programs.

Our program doesn't only teach you how to write a book – our team of coaches, developmental editors, copy editors, art directors, and marketing experts incubate you from having a book idea to being a published, bestselling author, ensuring that the book you create can actually make a difference in the world. Then we give you the training you need to use your book to make the difference in the world, or to create a business out of serving your readers.

ARE YOU READY TO MAKE A DIFFERENCE?

You've seen other people make a difference with a book. Now it's your turn. If you are ready to stop watching and start taking massive action, go to http://theauthorincubator.com/apply/.

"Yes, I'm ready!"

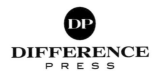

OTHER BOOKS BY DIFFERENCE PRESS

The Top 1% Life: The Real Estate Agent's Guide to Free Up Your Time, Build Your Business with Confidence, and Finally, Have a Life Outside of Sales!
by Kathleen Black

Get Back to Living: Navigating Through the Loss of Your Spouse
by Allison L. Brown

Stop Worrying about Your Anxious Child: How to Manage Your Child's Anxiety so You Can Finally Relax
by Tonya C. Crombie, Ph.D.

Become a Badass Rebel Runner: The Ultimate Guide to Being a Fit Mom without the Diet Bullshit
by Jane Elizabeth

From Borderline to Baseline: 9 Key Steps to Manage Your BPD and Start Loving Your Life
by Julie Ann Ford

Stop Draining Your Energy: The Movement Teacher's Guide to Attract Clients You Love
by Heather Glidden

Is This Sickness or an Energy Block?: Know the Difference and What to Do about It
by Amy Keast

Should I Leave My Relationship or Not?: The Smart Woman's Guide to a Clear Path Forward
by Karen Lin

Side Hustle to Main Hustle: The Corporate Woman's Guide to Full-Time Entrepreneurship
by Angel N. Livas

The Spiritual Entrepreneur: Quantum Leap Into Your Next Level of Impact and Abundance
by Angelina Lombardo

Invention Protection Strategies: Expose Your Intellectual Property and Fund Your Startup
by Cynthia Lombardo

Reverse Heart Disease Naturally: The Woman's Guide to Not Die before Your Time
by Laurie Morse

Know What You Want Next: Break Free of the 'I Don't Know' Trap and Love Your Life Again
by Kimberly Napier

Build Your Business with Social Media:
The Step-by-Step Guide to Create a Life You Love
by Gry Sinding

Should I Leave Nursing?: 7 Steps to Career Clarity
by Karen Beck Wade, Ph.D.